OM CANADA

*An Intimate Glimpse
at Yoga's Firsts*

VALERY PETRICH

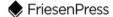 FriesenPress

Suite 300 - 990 Fort St
Victoria, BC, V8V 3K2
Canada

www.friesenpress.com

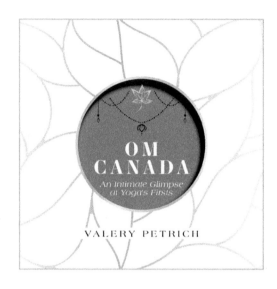

ISBN
978-1-5255-6523-6 (HARDCOVER)
978-1-5255-6524-3 (PAPERBACK)
978-1-5255-6525-0 (EBOOK)

Health & Fitness, Yoga

Distributed to the trade by The
Ingram Book Company

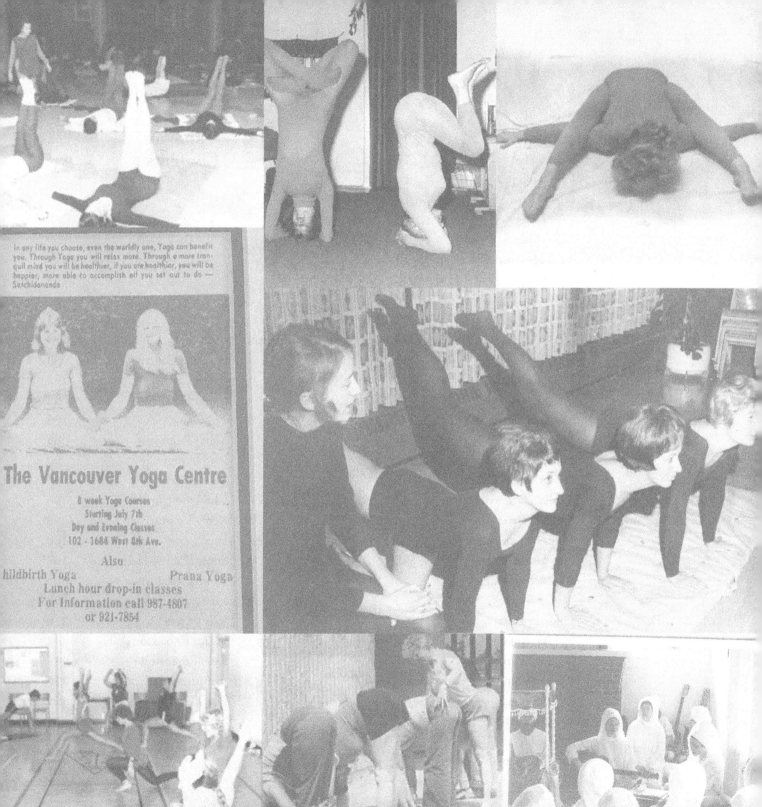

In any life you choose, even the worldly one, Yoga can benefit you. Through Yoga you will relax more. Through a more tranquil mind you will be healthier, if you are healthier, you will be happier, more able to accomplish all you set out to do — Satchidananda

The Vancouver Yoga Centre

8 week Yoga Courses
Starting July 7th
Day and Evening Classes
102 - 1688 West 8th Ave.

Also

hildbirth Yoga   Prana Yoga
Lunch hour drop-in classes
For information call 987-4807
or 921-7854

Table of Contents

Introduction

The first nudge to write this book happened when I was a guest at Rocklyn Ashram in Australia in 2013. At lunch one day a group of ladies at my table were passing around a book written by Australia's first yoga teacher, Roma Blair. There were some giggles about her trademark bouffant hairstyle and leopard tights. However, an earnest discussion followed about what Roma had done as the pioneer who introduced yoga to Australia through her TV series and the founder of International Yoga Teachers Association. What stood out for me was her exceptionally vivacious approach to life, even after suffering in a prisoner of war camp in Indonesia during World War II and subsequent health issues such as chronic stomach cramps. Known as the "mother of yoga" in Australia, Roma died at age ninety in 2013. I noted the awe and respect for Roma's contribution during the discussions and it made me think of our own icons in Canada.

The second nudge for this book was much later when I was hosting a yoga friend from Vancouver to teach at my yoga studio in Calgary. On the way to the airport she was talking about the good old days, when we used men's ties for straps and carpet underlay for yoga mats. I looked over at her and had a sharp realization of just how much time had passed since yoga had taken hold in Canada and how we both, now in our sixties, had witnessed a good chunk of it. Did the new generation, with its technical yoga wear and precision props, know there was a time without yoga belts, mats, or even studios? I asked if she had any pictures of herself from those days, recalling the afternoon in Australia when we were poring over Roma's book. I also thought of my first yoga teacher from 1975, Friedel Khattab, who was turning eighty-nine and who, in fact, had a picture of a young Roma on the wall in her bedroom. Who knew how much longer Friedel and others would be with us? I decided then and there, with absolute clarity, that the roots of yoga in Canada needed to be commemorated, even if it meant travelling from one end of the country to the other. So, that's exactly what I did.

Over the course of four years, I travelled from the West Coast to the Maritimes, interviewing the earliest known Canadian teachers. Some of them I already knew from many years of being a yoga teacher myself; others, I was led to.

I met Lois Morrison when I found out she attended my mother's church in Saskatoon. I found out about Ravi Ravindra while in a coffee shop in Halifax. I interviewed the world's oldest yoga teacher listed in the *Guiness Book of World Records* in her home in Orillia, Ontario, as we looked out at her backyard lake. I took a bus up to Auroraville, Ontario, to a property where the Yogastock retreats were held with Baba Hari Dass each year.

I visited sharp-as-a tack ninety-four-year-old Sister Elaine at her convent residence in Toronto, where she insisted her life was quite ordinary—but it wasn't. I met Marie Paulyn at her home in Toronto, and she was as much the picture of elegance at eighty-four as she was at thirty-five. Listening to Lillian Strauss's escapades in the Yukon made me chuckle. She truly did live in the bush, rolling her yoga mat out on a game reserve next to wild horses and other wildlife.

I met Guru Raj in her studio in Vancouver and she positively emanated joy. I left wanting to sign up for her training—and so it went. I regret that Joe Gnilke, age ninety and Swami Radha's earliest supporter, passed away a few weeks before our interview, but his wife kindly shared his diaries. Similar to Ruth Boutilier of Cape Breton, who passed away just weeks before my visit, but my long phone conversations with her had told me everything I needed to know about this extraordinary woman. Where the teacher had already died, I interviewed spouses, colleagues, students, sons, daughters, and grandchildren. I searched university archives and old newspapers. The good old YMCA and YWCA stand staunchly as the earliest supporters of yoga across Canada, but tracking records was not always easy because some had closed, some had burned down, and others had changed to women's shelters.

Everywhere I went, the hospitality was warm and teachers were supportive of my project. I was not prepared for the depth I heard in their life stories. The older the interviewee, the less they held back. Often, there were tears as people walked back through the chapters of their lives. I felt honoured that complete strangers would share the intimacies of their paths with me, until I realized that no yoga teacher is a stranger to the other.

For example, when I sought out legendary Kareen Zebroff, she poured her heart out and shared every aspect of her life, stopping just long enough to cook up a delicious shrimp lunch and then back to the table with memorabilia. She fell onto her bed with her clothes on at eight o'clock that night and went straight to sleep! From that experience and the many times with Kareen thereafter, I could see what made her a huge success. There was no bottom to her giving.

Although there are undoubtedly many other pioneers in Canada, I set out to find those who were distinct because they were the first—the first to introduce yoga in their city or town, the first to start a provincial association, the first to do a TV series, the first to start an ashram, the first to publish yoga books, and especially, the first to get in their cars in sub-zero temperatures to take yoga rural. I wanted to hear their stories. What motivated them? Where did they get their inspiration? Who taught them how to teach? How had yoga changed them? What personal suffering, such as that of Roma Blair, made them seek yoga?

I wanted to capture their unique contributions for all of us, but especially for today's yoga practitioners, so they could see that yoga was not always popular or even accepted. Practicing yoga was not cool. The subjects of this book were certainly not famous. There were no yoga rock stars. There was no such thing as a career in yoga, and mixing yoga and business was frowned upon. Some churches were reluctant to rent their basements to yoga teachers. There were accusations of cults and witchcraft. There were no neighborhood yoga studios and sometimes not even payment for teaching. Books were few. Accessibility to yoga was limited and mostly took place in major cities. Training often depended on visiting Americans.

Yoga's emergence in Canada began with a few survivors from World War II, surfaced with the counter-cultural movement of the 1960s, became fashionable in the 1970s, took a nosedive in popularity in the 1980s when the aerobic craze hit, and finally reached an unforeseen explosion in the late 1990s. This was in part due to celebrities like Madonna and Sting taking it up, but also because alternative health therapies were gaining their due, at last beginning to be endorsed by the medical profession. This last growth spurt of yoga in the West was unsurpassed by any other time in history. It was stunning for the fact that, within a few short years, it turned a centuries-old patriarchal tradition on its head for now being spearheaded mostly by women. As the number of practitioners in the US doubled and then doubled again, the pioneers were spotlighted. They were now recognized as change agents in this evolutionary leap.

There are certain characteristics in these teachers. Often motivated by a strong spiritual awakening, or a desire to have one, they sometimes embarked on a spiritual inquiry due to a painful life event—loss of a loved one, lingering trauma from war, an unexpected medical diagnosis, a "nervous breakdown," a hidden addiction, a painful back problem, and so on. For others, the spiritual path was chosen for them as they experienced a spontaneous *kundalini* awakening, received *shaktiput* through a master or, through a twist of fate, were born a visionary with psychic ability.

Almost all of them were attracted to yoga for its health-giving benefits. They found the overall quality of their lives improved with yoga practice and became inextricably drawn toward sharing it with others.

A few took a leap of faith when they found their guru, often accompanied by a feeling of familiarity. They often had premonitions and a strong sense of guidance when these encounters happened, not unlike saints, sages, and mystics. They made a choice to listen to that calling and they led their lives in service to it. I'm sure it was not easy.

These teachers and leaders possessed high levels of compassion for others—in short, they were and are humanitarians. They were and are ordinary people, just like you and me, but became extraordinary by listening to their intuition and following their spiritual paths. They left a meaningful mark on the lives of countless others through their generosity and innovation.

Yoga in Canada emerged from a barren landscape as these people established the roots of yoga and meditation for you and me. They did so quietly and humbly. Let their stories inspire you to kindle the next chapter in your life.

Part 1
Survivors

These remarkable leaders were not only the first teachers in Canada, they also had a shared experience of trauma and pain from World War II. Full of optimism for a life of peace, they chose a fresh start in Canada. They used the tools of yoga artfully, finding that the practice in all its forms calmed their nervous systems, improved their health, and gave them a sense of mastery over their lives. Of those still alive that I interviewed, I couldn't help but notice they displayed a strong sense of purpose in their lives as well as an elevated sense of gratitude—perhaps because of their pasts. Through their transformational experience of triumph over tragedy, they became uniquely equipped to help others. Some of them were the first Canadian yoga teachers to work with veterans. They taught yoga nidra (yogic sleep), meditation, and yogic breathing for those veterans experiencing battle fatigue and shell shock (now called post-traumatic stress disorder or PTSD). My observation of those I interviewed is that they naturally fell into their roles. They showed willingness to heal the scars of the past and bring joy into each day, and I attribute this resilience to their practice. Their admirable qualities set a humanitarian tone as they laid the foundation for yoga in Canada.

Franz Achatz

Born Germany, 1913; died Toronto,
Ontario, 1982

Helen Achatz

Born Germany, year unknown; died Toronto,
Ontario, 1989

Franz and Helen Achatz immigrated to Canada
from Germany in the early 1950s. Products of
Hitler's push for physical perfection, Franz and
Helen Achatz had become successful ballet dancers
in their native Germany during the Nazi era.

Once in Canada, they applied the same perfec-
tionism and intensity to their newfound passion
for yoga. They easily mastered the poses, but were
especially drawn to the esotericism of yoga philosophy that they practiced and taught in the Sivananda
method. They were the second to open a yoga studio
in Toronto, after John and Tinie Gollop, which
became Toronto's longest running studio. Opening
at 935 Bloor Street in 1970, they initially named it
the Yoga and Ballet Centre, then changed the name
to Yoga Centre Toronto. They trained many teachers
who are some of Ontario's most senior teachers today.
Admired for his inquiring, keen mind and passion
for philosophy, Franz became active on the lecture
circuit. So strong was their love of establishing a yoga
community that they were considered by many to be
the "mother and father" of yoga in Ontario.

Long-time student Lila Ostermann became Yoga
Centre Toronto's director in 1971, with Marion
Harris as co-director. In 1974, the centre was relo-
cated to 2428 Yonge Street, with subsequent direc-
tors including Joyce Hawkeye, Yvonne McKinley,
Bala Jaison, and Wendy Cole. At time of printing,
Marlene Mawhinney was at the helm.

The Achatzes' love of gardening and flowers led
them to purchase a farm in Eganville, Ontario,
which became a popular retreat for yoga trainings,
including teacher training certification programs.
They were legendary for their many meals of fellowship around the large, farm-sized table, sharing
discourse on yoga and metaphysics, reincarnation,
and evolution.

Says Bala Jaison of those times together: "Franz
and Helen were remarkable people. They had profound wisdom. They were, as referred to in metaphysics, very evolved souls. They had an uncanny
ability to 'read' people—what they were thinking,
what they felt, what they needed. This helped them
guide their students to experience new avenues
of consciousness.

"They took me under their wing and I lived
with them for three months and received personal
training. Franz taught me yoga every morning—he
encouraged perfection in each posture, and some
of the asanas were really intense. Weekends were
time for reflection on work done during the week.
There are no words to express the gratitude I feel for
them—what I learned from them ended up guiding
me into my professional life as a psychotherapist."

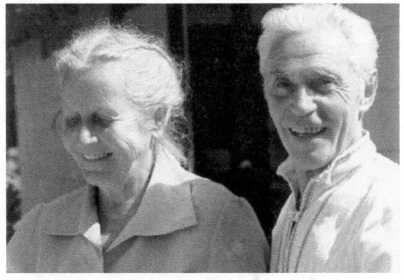

Helen and Franz Achatz, founders, Yoga Centre Toronto

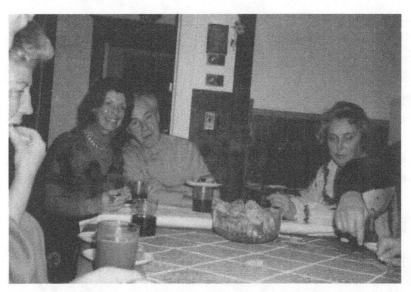

Marie, Franz, and Helen, Eganville, Ontario, farm

John Gollop

Born Niagara-on-the-Lake, Ontario, 1922; died
Etobicoke, Ontario, 2000

Tinie Gollop

Born Amsterdam, Netherlands, 1922; died
Etobicoke, Ontario, 2015

John and Tinie Gollop are legends for both their
enduring love story and their distinction as the ear-
liest-known yoga pioneers in Canada. They started
teaching yoga in Niagara-on-the-Lake in 1946, and
together opened the first-known yoga studio in
Canada, in 1956.

John was a Canadian soldier, serving in Holland
during World War II, and Tinie was a Dutch native
and budding ballerina at the Amsterdam Opera
House. Tinie met John while working in the Dutch
resistance and when the war ended in 1945, they
married in Amsterdam.

During a short stay in England, John attended a
trauma recovery program for veterans that included
yoga and meditation. Finding it a great help, he
briefly studied yoga with an unnamed Asian master
before returning to Canada with Tinie in 1946. They
took up residence at John's birthplace of Niagara-on-
the-Lake, where Tinie founded her own ballet school
and also taught yoga along with John.

John worked at Magneto Electric and occasionally took jobs teaching yoga on cruise ships. His real
interest, however, was teaching yoga and meditation
to his fellow veterans to relieve symptoms associ-
ated with PSTD. John registered the earliest known
Canadian non-profit yoga organization in 1950,
calling it the Yoga Society of Canada. He and Tinie
continued to teach in schools and centres before
moving to Toronto, where they built Ontario's first
known yoga studio onto their house in Etobicoke.

The spiritual strength the Gollops drew from
yoga helped them through the loss of their only
child, Gloria. They are legendary for their compassion as teachers, dedicated to easing the suffering
they saw around them. As founding members of the
Federation of Ontario Yoga Teachers, they laid the
foundation for yoga in Ontario. They hosted workshops and presenters to improve the quality of yoga
teachers. They became close friends with fellow early
yoga teachers Franz and Helen Achatz.

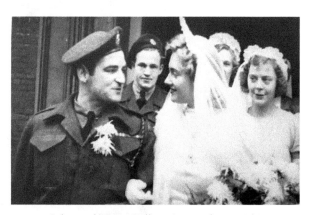

John and Tinie Gollop, Amsterdam, 1945

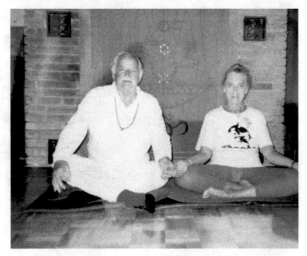

John and Tinie Gollop, Islington, Ontario studio

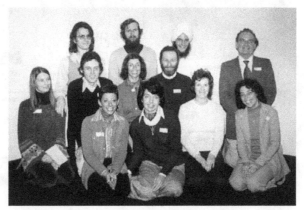

Federation of Ontario Yoga Teachers, FOYT, 1974
Back row: Danny Johnson, Chris Laidler, Ted Steiner (Gurtej Singh), John Gollop,
Middle row: Joyce Hawkeye, Patrick McCaffrey, Marie Paulyn, Barry Dykes
Front row: Bala Jaison, Marion Harris, Yvonne McKinley, Chris Byers

ROTARY

Yoga master visits the Krugersdorp club

By Barry West

NOT EVEN imminent departure on a Jumbo Jet could prevent a well-known Canadian yoga master from addressing Krugersdorp Rotarians recently, and within minutes of the completion of his speech, he was speeding off to Jan Smuts airport.

John Gollop of Toronto has been a yoga exponent for 40 years and is one of the leading men in this field in Canada. His recent visit to South Africa, where he renewed his friendship with local businessman Arthur Carter, was just a holiday but on being asked to address the Rotary club he readily agreed.

Unfortunately the only time available was just four hours before his return to Canada.

John served in the Canadian forces during World War II, was captured in Europe and ended up in a prisoner of war camp. When war ended he found himself in Holland and stayed on in the country, eventually marrying a Dutch girl.

He made his way back to Canada via London, and it was here that he met an Indian swami who introduced him to yoga.

John said: "I had nervous troubles after being cooped up in the POW camp and yoga really helped me get over those problems. When I returned to Canada I used what I had learned to help other soldiers, who suffered the same type of nervous complaints, get over their pain through yoga".

Since then John has been on television and gives classes each week to professional and business people, young and old, men and women.

"It surprises some people that I have so many men in my classes but, with the amount of business people who suffer burn-out because of the stresses entailed in their jobs, yoga seems to help them relax. Another reason why people attend my classes is the incidence of back trouble, yoga helps immensely to alleviate this".

Because yoga is not competitive people in any age group adapt well to the regime and as John pointed out: "You are never too young or old for yoga it really gives you boundless energy".

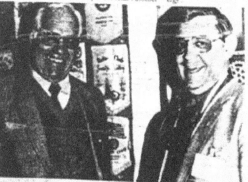

Colin Steyn the president of Krugersdorp Rotary Club, inducts new members Martin Ellis into the club.

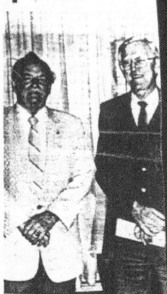

John Gollop and Arthur Carter . . . friends many years.

John Gollop speaks in South Africa

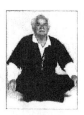

John Gollop

John has taught Yoga since 1946. John and his wife Tinie, founded the Yoga Society of Canada, Islington, Ontario, where both taught for many years.

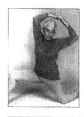

Lila Osterman

Lila is one of the most highly respected and well-known names in Yoga in Canada. She is the founder of The Yoga Centre in Toronto and has over thirty years experience in her study and teaching of Yoga. Lila travels throughout Canada and the U.S. presenting workshops on Yoga and related topics and concepts.

Tinie Gollop

A classical ballet dancer, who also studied Law, met John shortly after the war in her native Holland. They married - he taught her Yoga, and she taught him Ballet! Their "Yoga-ballets" became so popular that other companies emulated them. Tinie has danced and taught Yoga internationally. John and Tinie are great-grandparents.

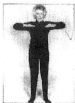

Penny Sanderson

Penny began her Yoga career in 1971 after an acute attack of arthritis left her immobile. She was able to take over teaching the class three months later. She studied under Marie Paulyn and has taught Yoga since 1972.

Margaret Siedel

Since 1966 Margaret has been involved in such Yogic activities as teaching, helping to run the Achatz Yoga Retreat Centre, and spells with Algonquin College and Renfrew Board of Education, often teaching as many as eight classes per week. Margaret was known as the "travelling" Yoga teacher, with a weekly TV show in Pembroke, Ottawa on Yoga, herbs and alternative lifestyle disciplines, and in 1976 built a "huge" herb garden, and is still helping people with herbs.

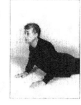

Sheila Haslam

Sheila joined FOYT in 1976 and is a former Board Member and President. She has been practising Yoga for over 30 years.

Muriel Church

Muriel refers to herself as 71 years-young, and her Yoga career has spanned almost three decades. Her philosophy of life is: "Education is a daily procedure - we are all taking studies at the University of Daily Living. Graduation date unknown! To be sure, I have been on the YOGA adventure all of my life."

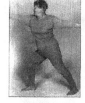

Edna Wright

Edna's long career in Yoga started in 1971. "One summer I went to the Howard Kent school in the U.K., and was lucky enough to meet Wilfred Clark, founder of the British Wheel of Yoga. We became firm friends, and through him I took the exam and gained my certificate through "The All India Board of Yoga". I became a teacher in the early 70's."

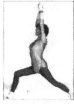

Marie Paulyn

In 1972 Marie founded the School of Hatha and Raja Yoga in Toronto, and in 1975 introduced her first Yoga Teacher Training course. Marie is a founding member of FOYT, an active member of the Association for Humanistic Psychology, and the International Association of Yoga Therapists.

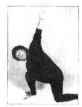

Ola Manuel

Ola was introduced to Yoga early in 1966 by Dr. Bena Nelson, whilst attending a seminar for Fitness Directors of the YWCA Canada, and in 1970 introduced Yoga to fitness classes at the YWCA in Niagara Falls. She now shares a partnership with Regis Woodward at their Yoga for Fitness Centre at the Loretto Retreat Centre in Niagara Falls.

Rachel Kanner

Rachel's introduction to Yoga came in 1960, in Jerusalem, when, as a counter activity to a very heavy study schedule, she started to take Yoga classes. Back in Toronto in 1981, studied under John Gallop, and graduating from Marie Paulyn's teacher training in 1977. Rachel was Treasurer for many years, and was largely responsible for bringing FOYT out of the red to its present strong financial position.

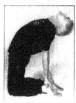

Regis Woodward

In 1973, he became the first male YWCA staff member and the only male Yoga teacher in the Niagara District. In 1975, recognizing the needs of the disabled and their handicaps, and together with Ola Manuel, whom he describes as, "My teacher and partner" Regis helped form Yoga for the Handicapped, which was actually the beginnings of the Yoga for Fitness Centre, circa. 1979.

FOYT 25th anniversary calendar, 1999

Friedel Khattab

Born Heisenberg, Germany, 1923; died Edmonton, Alberta, 2015

Friedel Khattab was the longest-serving yoga teacher and the first yoga businesswoman in Alberta, and she established the first yoga school in Alberta.

She is a legend, but it also needs to be said that she was formidable. This is likely due to her early years. As a young woman living in Hitler's Germany, she was strongly encouraged in gymnastics and later studied physical therapy. She spent four years in the German army and became a stickler about detail and precision, qualities that were to last all her life. When she became a yoga teacher, it wasn't uncommon to hear her add (half playfully), "And that's an order!"

Due to recurring pneumonia, she was released from the army and reassigned to caretaking children in the countryside during the last years of World War II. The years of hunger in Germany also took a toll on Friedel, and she developed macular degeneration in her eyes. Thus, she wore her signature sunglasses while teaching throughout her life.

Friedel took an enthusiastic interest in yogic breathing as a way to alleviate her lung condition. She liked to tell the story of helping a Jewish war survivor pass his medical for entry into the US by taking him into the mountain air for two months of rigorous yogic breathing instruction. Ultimately, he passed his test.

After the war, she lived and worked in London, where she sought out yoga classes at the local YWCA. When she met and married her husband, Sharif, in 1955, they moved to his home in Cairo, where they stayed for eleven years.

Immersed in a thriving yoga community in Cairo, Friedel took classes from Yogi Shakti of Calcutta and the Indian ambassador Ape Pant, who taught her the sun salutation series. She studied meditation with Maharishi Mahesh Yogi when he arrived in 1963. Friends often met at her house to practice. During that time, Friedel had three children successively, so squeezing in yoga practice was more than a simple trick.

At the end of the Israeli-Egyptian war in 1967, President Nasser gave an edict that anyone so choosing to could leave Egypt, but had to do so immediately. With $411 and five suitcases, the Khattab family made their way to Canada, settling in Edmonton. Friedel immediately started teaching at the YWCA. When her class sizes ballooned to over fifty people, she left the Y to rent her own space in a church and library, and there she stayed for years. She insisted on people signing up for ten-week sessions, claiming that was the best way to experience results. Friedel had a way of telling people what to do, and they did it!

When she founded Friedel Khattab's School of Yoga in 1970, she certified the first four teachers in Alberta. She was undisputedly Alberta's first yoga businesswoman, taking yoga from an era of donations in a basket to a paycheque. She also placed ads regularly in *The Edmonton Journal*, negotiating editorials about her work in return.

Having a lifelong fascination with the movements of the human body and always wanting to learn something new, Friedel was often on a plane to meet a new "master." She would memorize everything in an impeccable manner and return home to teach it. She trained with some of the greats and in all corners of the globe.

Friedel taught at the Yasodhara Ashram in Kootenay Bay, British Columbia, in summers, taking her daughters with her. She and Swami Radha developed a special friendship based on a shared past in wartime Germany. When interviewed, Friedel recounted the time she travelled with Swami Radha to celebrate the swami's seventy-fifth birthday in California. The swami took Friedel shopping to buy her a new dress—during her reminiscence, Friedel's face took on the softness of a child. She praised Swami Radha highly, saying, "She was very smart and she had a purpose."

As Friedel gained increasing respect as a yoga expert, she accepted invitations to teach across Canada, the US, and Costa Rica, always inviting them back to teach in Edmonton.

One of her last trainings was at the Yoga Studio of Calgary at age ninety, where she taught a lymphatic cleanse series she'd learned from a Tibetan master. The attendees raved about the results and embraced her warmly, not knowing it would be the last time they would be in the company of this remarkable woman.

Friedel passed away in 2016 at age ninety-one of a stroke. She was still actively training teachers at the Yoga for Today studio in Edmonton until she fell ill. One yoga teacher described her this way: "She will be sorely missed. She was a tough-love mother with the soul of a kitten." Her legacy lives on in the over 1,000 diverse teachers she has trained, many of them now spread across Canada.

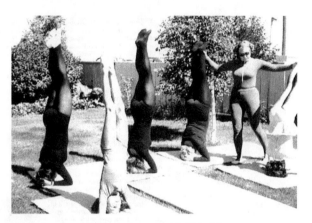

Backyard yoga with Friedel

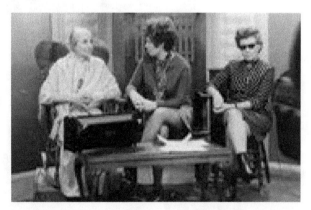

Swami Radha and Friedel interview, CBC 1971

FRIEDEL KHATTAB:

NO ORDINARY YOGA TEACHER

by Jean Burgess

Yoga classes! Workshops! Teacher training! Can one Yoga teacher offer all these? Yes. Friedel Khattab s School of Yoga established in Edmonton, Alberta in 1968 does just that.

Beginning in September, for seven months of each year Khattab teaches a combination of the traditional Indian Hatha Yoga, and the Okido technique — a remedial Oriental Yoga developed by Masahiro Oki of Mishima, Japan. The Oki System is very highly regarded as a means to achieve weight reduction and physical fitness. Then when classes are over in May, Friedel travels around the world, to an Ashram to discover new Yoga techniques, or a treatment centre seeking remedial methods.

"Years ago there was a surge of Swamis coming to Canada to conduct workshops," says Friedel. "Now, not only are these people getting old, their techniques have been learned and spread. Today, with qualified Canadian and US teachers, the Swamis are no longer needed."

It was in 1979 that Friedel journeyed to Japan to work for her teacher s certificate in the Okido System. There were three groups of 65 students at the Ashram. Classes, scheduled from 5:00 a.m. to 7:00 p.m., ran for six weeks. One morning another student in the course suffered an epileptic seizure. Friedel went to the assistance of her classmate.

"Will you teach us what you know about epilepsy?" she was asked later that day. So, making notes that night, and with the help of an excellent interpreter, Friedel taught the class about care for epileptics. They valued her contribution: half the cost of the course was refunded. As for herself, she was captivated by the therapeutic effectiveness and astonishing results of Master Oki s approach.

What marks the beginning of a yoga teacher?

Friedel Khattab trained as a physical education instructor in Germany. Then for four and a half years worked as a physiotherapist in camps and hospitals during World War II. In the summer of 1947 Germany lay in ruins. At the same time the United States had just opened its doors to immigrants from Europe — if they were healthy. An old doctor at the newly set up clinic looked hard at Friedel and said, "There could be a chance ... deep breathing, ribcage expansion, hold the breath as long as possible and exhale completely. You will get all the fresh air you need."

In the foothills of the Bavarian Alps, fresh air was about the only thing in abundance that summer of '47. Just by chance an elderly mountaineering

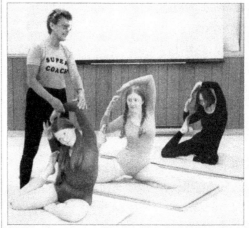

Friedel Khattab trains teachers in the intricate pidgeon pose.

Friedel Khattab, *Foresight Magazine*, 1987

Yoga seminar, Edmonton

Gerda Krebs

Born Prussia, 1931 –

While growing up in Hitler's Germany, young Gerda was trained in gymnastics by her father. Like many Germans in that time, she was encouraged to excel in a physical discipline. The ravages of the World War and the loss of her mother in a bombing in Germany were painful for Gerda, and she carried that pain to Canada when she immigrated with her husband Heinz in 1952.

When she saw an ad in *The Edmonton Journal* for yoga in 1967, something spoke to her. Perhaps this yoga thing would allow her do the exercise she loved so much but also give her peace of mind? When she started classes with Friedel Khattab at St. Augustine Church, she had a profound experience in *savasana* (relaxation). It felt so peaceful. She knew she was where she needed to be, so she signed up for the first teacher training program offered by Friedel in 1970.

Gerda began teaching up to fifteen classes per week in Sherwood Park, Alberta, including classes for people with migraines and back problems. Representing the Yoga Association of Alberta, she went on to teach in many small towns in that province, travelling by bus or small plane to remote locations. Before long, she was approached to host a yoga TV series, which Shaw launched in 1975 and became the longest-running in Canada.

Much of "Yoga Fits In" was filmed at her acreage, giving it a warm, inviting feel. The series ran for twenty-five years, reaching many who otherwise had no access to yoga. Gerda laughingly remembers those days: "My 'gym' suits were specially made for me by the producer of the show. I used to teach yoga on a bearskin rug and someone called in to complain, so we had to scrap that!"

She also recalls resistance to yoga by some churches in those days. When a couple of individuals went door to door to dissuade people from attending yoga classes with her, Gerda made up her mind to educate people about what yoga really was. "Yoga is a philosophy. It will make you a better Christian. Yoga philosophy teaches us to do good deeds," says Gerda. Her frequent articles in the Sherwood Newspaper were informative and full of encouragement for beginners.

Gerda didn't travel much for additional trainings. "If my husband wanted to go to Canadian Tire on a Saturday and wanted me to accompany him, I would go, even though I didn't want to," she recalls. "We were partners and that's how I stayed married. Yoga is what I wanted to do, and he supported me." Heinz passed away in 2002.

Gerda has trained many teachers; true to her mentor Friedel, she encourages trainees to jump in and start teaching right away, following a firm curriculum.

Her admirers planted a tree in her name in Sherwood Park when she turned seventy. She did not slow down, however. Well into her late eighties, Gerda still actively trains teachers at Yoga for Today in Edmonton. She claims one of her secrets to youthfulness is a glass of warm water with lemon juice first thing in the morning, which she has done for over thirty years. Her attitude is summed up in one of her favourite quotes: "The one who lives content with little possesses everything."

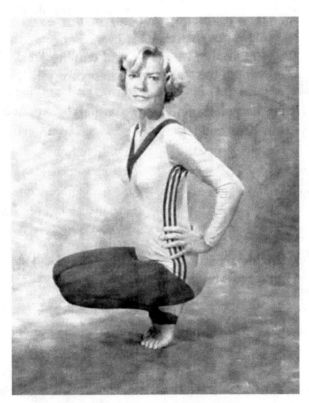

Gerda Krebs taping 'Yoga Fits'

Axel Molema

Born Assenede, Belgium, 1941 –

Axel grew up in a Holland that was being torn apart by World War II. He immigrated to Woodbridge, Ontario, at ten years old, carrying with him memories of first-hand deprivation from the war and a particular sensitivity to suffering. This sensitivity was to shape his life in becoming a heartfelt, spiritual teacher.

Axel became a full-time yoga teacher and has taught over 40,000 classes in a career spanning over five decades.

Axel began as senior piping draftsman, but life took a turn when a Dutch colleague introduced him to yoga. In 1966, he discovered the Sivananda Vedanta Centre on Bloor Street in Toronto. There, he met the centre's director, Swami Vishnudevananda, as well as pioneers Franz and Helen Achatz, who founded the Yoga Centre Toronto. Befriended by Franz and Helen, he became one of their most ardent students. When Franz gave a talk, Axel would demonstrate the poses and Axel started to sub a few of Franz's classes in the Toronto area.

Axel quit his day job in 1970. It was crystal clear to him that his path was to serve others and create sacred space, and he never wavered from it. He bought dozens of books written by Swami Sivananda and studied at the Sivananda Ashram at Val Morin, Quebec.

Despite Axel's professed skepticism of gurus, Swami Sivananda of India became the most influential teacher over his lifetime. Says Axel: "I could never go to India—I was a householder, married with children. If you can't be with an enlightened being, the best thing to do is acquire their books. I happen to be very study-oriented and I applied it. I chose the Sivananda tradition because it is a sacred tradition from the Shankaracharya period, and I feel he is the widest-known, most reputable guru. I teach a synthesis of Karma Yoga, Bhakti Yoga, asana, and Jnana Yoga practice. It all bears fruit when you sustain the practice." Axel became a vegetarian and stopped alcohol altogether.

Axel's teaching history includes sessions at York University, the University of Toronto, Seneca College, and North York and Mount Sinai hospitals. Never interested in being a studio owner, he always rented space, primarily from churches. He has also conducted highly popular spring and fall retreats at Lake Simcoe and Jackson's Point, Ontario, for many years.

Says Axel: "Karma will determine how much longer I teach. Retirement doesn't appeal to me, so I will teach as long as I am healthy. I strive to teach meaningful classes, offering my long-term students a better life on mental, spiritual, and physical levels. A psychic told me at age twenty-five that my reincarnations were a monk in India, one in China, and one in Europe as a Roman Catholic priest. It all influences who I am now! Yogananda states that the abilities you have at birth are 75 percent from previous incarnations and 25 percent from what we acquire from parents, school, environment, and so on."

Axel continues to teach in the Toronto area. His teaching style is uniquely Axel. He chooses to teach without props or corrections. He sits cross-legged at the head of the class, giving occasional profound spiritual contemplations quietly, like drops of rain on a still evening. His approach invites his students to use each pose as a spiritual inquiry into how they live their lives. The loyalty and love from students who have been with him up to forty years show that it works.

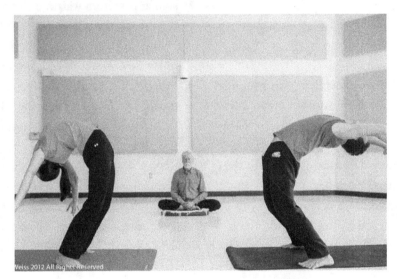

Axel Molema, 50 years teaching. Photo: Bryan Weiss

Adelinde (Lila) Ostermann

Born Germany, 1919; died Salt Spring Island, British Columbia, 2010

Known as Lila, Adelinde Ostermann was a young woman when World War II overtook Europe. She was trained as a Red Cross nurse and stationed near the Russian front, where she witnessed brutal devastation. Her boyfriend was subsequently killed in the war and this sadness stayed with her.

When she immigrated to Canada in 1953 with a young son, Matthias, it was full of hope for a new, pain-free life. But it didn't turn out that way—at least not in the beginning. Lila was using alcohol and cigarettes to dull her pain, and a brush with cancer finally convinced her to seek meaning in her life and turn it around. When she found yoga through the Sivananda method, she found a path that helped her embrace good health, joy, and community. Experiencing nothing short of a rebirth, she became a passionate teacher. Lila's poignant story is one of triumph over tragedy—her sole purpose became to help ease suffering in others.

For the next forty years, Lila gained a solid reputation for training quality teachers from coast to coast. She was also the first Canadian to be appointed director of the teacher training program at Kripalu Ashram in Pennsylvania, which she did successfully for eight years.

In 1970, Lila found Franz and Helen Achatz, the early founders of Yoga Centre Toronto. They shared a similar past from wartime Germany and Lila became their devoted student and close friend. After furthering her teacher training with well-known Indra Devi in Mexico, she returned home and assumed directorship of YTC, succeeding Franz and Helen, who had moved to a farm in Eganville, Ontario.

Lila was a dynamo. To boost the yoga community, she brought in well-known names, such as Swami Radha, Swami Vishnudevananda, Marcia Moore, and many others. She also established many satellite locations with teachers around the Toronto area.

During this time she experienced two painful relationships. Her first love interest took her car and her money; one night she followed him and knocked on his door—his wife answered and said they had been married for eleven years. Her second love interest turned out to be gay. Said one teacher who worked with her in the 1970s, "She was a good soul, and people exploited her—she was desperate to be loved and accepted."

When she met Yogi Amrit Desai and was introduced to the Kripalu style of "meditation in motion," she was newly inspired. A new depth and sensitivity came into her teaching, and, after her painful love life, she embraced it. She moved to the Kripalu ashram in Pennsylvania in 1974 and became a popular teacher known for her compassion. She travelled to India to meet founder Amrit's Desai's guru, Swami Kripalvananda. He bestowed her with the name *Lila*, which means "cosmic energy." In 1976, Lila was asked to assist in the creation of the upgraded Kripalu Ashram as well as become director of their teacher training program.

In 1984, at age sixty-five, Lila returned to Canada to live for a few quiet years in a small ashram in Ontario. In the early 1990s, she started visiting Salt Spring Island to teach for the ten-day annual retreats with Baba Hari Dass, and in 2003, she moved there permanently. Over time she slowly withdrew from teaching due to a heart attack, and drew solace from tending her much-loved garden.

Lila once said, "I want to die repeating *japa* on my lips." Surrounded by a group of loyal students until the end, she died in 2010 at age ninety. Only one year earlier, she had lost her only child, Matthias, a well-known artist and author, to AIDS.

Lila touched many people. Those who knew her describe her as someone who "exuded the joy of a child that belied the early painful years she had endured." She remains a Canadian yoga icon for her tireless work giving workshops and lectures, training teachers, and leading thousands to a healthier, more spiritually fulfilling and joyful life from coast to coast.

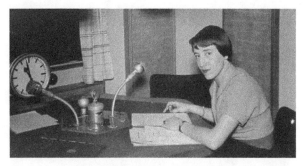

Lila Ostermann Germany,1941

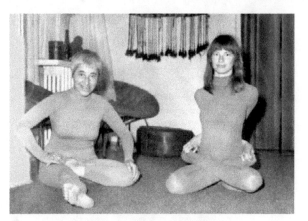

Lila Ostermann and Joyce Hawkeye, 1973

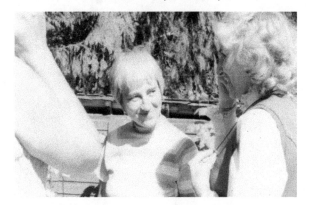

Lila and Swami Radha at Yasodhara Ashram

Part 2
Searchers

These pioneers sought to deepen what was an obscure practice in the 1960s and '70s. The esotericism of yoga appealed to them and guided them to find answers. Some of their sons and daughters described them as "ahead of their time" as they went against the established norm.

The people in this chapter aren't people that woke up every day and said, "I am going to radically transform the world today by leaving pearls of wisdom for future generations," but that is, indeed, what happened—little by little, as they uncovered whatever they could find on yoga and shared it with others. They were able later to look back over their shoulders and say, "Wow, I did that!"

When I interviewed these seekers I found them to be as diverse as Canada itself—from quiet Prairie people, to West Coast hippie types, to hearty Cape Breton souls. They all paved the way for our flourishing yoga communities today. They sought out what few books there were, and practiced along with Kareen Zebroff's TV series when it came out in 1970. Later, they waited for their glossy monthly *Yoga Journal* from San Francisco to arrive in their mailboxes and tell them where to find teachers—mostly Americans who felt like our older brothers and sisters. They started provincial yoga associations as a way to bring likeminded people together, and mailed newsletters to connect people who were long distances apart. They figured things out by keenly watching what other countries were doing, such as the well-established British Wheel of Yoga. Here and there, the first workshops and conferences emerged. They supported each other to be confident teachers long before there were certifying bodies, often quipping, "It is the students that certify the teacher."

Little did they know they were charting an evolutionary path that would take yoga out of church basements to become a presence in every neighbourhood. As a testament to yoga's youthfulness, many of these pioneers became "lifers" who were still passionate about their practices fifty years later. They did what they did because they loved yoga, and most were not even particularly concerned about legacy—it was practice for its own sake. In so doing, they created the drumbeat that many others would follow.

Sheri Berkowitz

Born Winnipeg, Manitoba, 1942 –

Sheri's first exposure to yoga was seeing her grandmother do yoga on TV in Los Angeles along with well-known American Richard Hittleman's TV show. Later, she was gifted the book *The Complete Illustrated Book of Yoga*, written by Swami Vishnudevananda. In 1973, her cousin invited her to take a class at the home of Winnipeg yoga teacher Barbara Preston, and Sheri jumped at the chance.

The experience sparked a path for Sheri that was to span almost fifty years as a student, teacher, mentor, and one of Canada's yoga leaders. Sheri's guiding hand was evident from the earliest days of the yoga scene in Winnipeg.

She started teaching and was part of a small, eclectic group who were passionate and spiritually curious about yoga. They met regularly at the YMCA and started with the customary Sivananda chanting for half hour before each meeting. This led to the formation of the Yoga Teachers Association of Manitoba in 1974, of which Sheri was a founding member. They established guidelines for teacher trainings and brought in expert teachers such as Americans Rama Vernon, Jean Couch, Judith Lasater, and Marcia Moore.

Sheri was inspired by Swami Mahadevananda's visits from the Sivananda Centre in Montreal. Says Sheri: "He was a marvelous and inspirational teacher who worked us seriously and did a great deal of questioning so that we could think our way through the teachings."

In 1979, Sheri immersed herself in the daily rigorous style alongside local Indian practitioners at the Iyengar Institute in Pune, India. Her adventurous spirit also took her to the Rajneesh Ashram to see author and teacher Bhagwan Shree Rajneesh (Osho), who later became a controversial figure in Oregon, US. Sheri returned three more times to study in Pune. She later studied at the Iyengar Yoga Institute of San Francisco in 1984-85, and then shared her knowledge with the Winnipeg yoga community. She practiced weekly with her long-time friend and teacher Karen Fletcher.

Sheri played a large role in growing the community in Winnipeg. As a senior teacher, she helped launch Yoga Centre Winnipeg in 1986. Says fellow teacher Hart Lazer: "Sheri was really supportive. She lent the studio thousands of dollars to set up, and at one point she paid my way to do training with Ramanand Patel in the US. She encouraged us to charge for yoga and be professional. I learned a lot from her."

Sheri's reputation spread beyond Winnipeg as she accepted invitations to train teachers in other cities. One of those cities was Kenora, Ontario, where

Laurie Jo Lindroos hosts a thriving community today. "I began yoga after the loss of my child. Grace led the way, and I met Sheri, whose light, inspiration, and knowledge opened new doors for me," says Laurie Jo.

Sheri left Winnipeg for Salt Spring Island, British Columbia, where she started a yoga studio and permaculture farm. She now splits her time between Victoria, British Columbia, and California, where she occasionally teaches at the Yoga Centre of Palm Desert with Holly Hoffman. Sheri recently resigned from the executive board of the Canadian Iyengar Yoga Association after serving for many years. Her influence still lives on in Winnipeg, where she is remembered for being an early guiding hand in all things yoga.

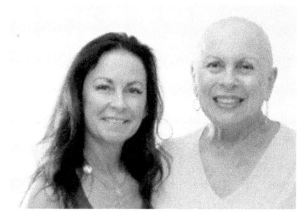

Sheri Berkowitz (right) with Holly Hoffman

Ruth Boutilier

Born Glace Bay, Nova Scotia, 1935; died Sidney, Nova Scotia, 2018

While growing up in Cape Breton, Nova Scotia, Ruth first saw yoga watching TV in 1954 as California fitness guru Paul Bragg demonstrated sun salutations on the iconic Ed Sullivan show. When she later found Jesse Stearn's book *Yoga, Youth and Reincarnation,* her interest was further kindled. Ruth taught from books in the mid-1960s, later brushing up her skills when Kareen Zebroff debuted on TV. When she convinced the local YMCA to hold a class to gauge interest in 1970, the response was overwhelming—248 people showed up and paid the YMCA one dollar per head. Cape Breton had found their yoga instructor, and Ruth would remain their beloved teacher for the next fifty years.

Ruth became an icon in Nova Scotia as the first lady of yoga. She did a yoga show on cable TV in the 1980s, taught ten weekly classes, and wrote a weekly yoga column that ran in the *Cape Breton Post.*

Ruth was very clear early on that she had a calling. In her words: "In 1971, I took the phonebooks for Montreal and Toronto and there was nothing under yoga. So I said a prayer every night that I could somehow find a way to study yoga. I said, 'Lord if you show me the way, I will do all of the work.'"

This passionate pursuit led her to walk through the doors of the Sivananda Vedanta Centre in Montreal, and eventually to earn certification in the Sivananda tradition at their ashram in Val Morin, Quebec.

She was a graduate of the first teacher training program at the Kripalu Ashram, at that time situated in an old barn near Reading, Pennsylvania. It was here she met fellow Canadian Friedel Khattab of Edmonton, and they became fast friends, conducting workshops in each other's cities. They were similar personalities—fiery and feisty and single-minded in their purpose.

Ruth spent many summers volunteer teaching for Marilyn Rossner's popular children's camp at the Sivananda Ashram in Val Morin. Children and youth, often with special needs, came from all over the world for yoga therapy.

Ruth's weekly classes included the MS Society, Seaview nursing homes, and the addiction centre, where the director came to her class and stayed for years. She taught men's and children's classes and felt especially rewarded by her classes at the Canadian Institute for the Blind in Glace Bay. She taught at the Holy Trinity Catholic Church in Sydney Mines, Nova Scotia, where her student Francis MacNeil, at age ninety-two, recalled fondly: "I came to classes in 1970 with my two daughters as well as my two daughters-in-law. Next to us were always three Notre Dame nuns. All of us practiced headstands and shoulder stands, coached by our high-energy teacher. We loved every minute of it. Would you believe I still do yoga?"

Ruth never cared about the money part of yoga—she was passionate that as many people as possible discovered its benefits, and this only enhanced her popularity. Said Ruth in 2018: "I still charge five dollars for my class. I plan on raising my fee when they make a six-dollar bill!"

Appreciative of her full life until the end, Ruth said, "I believe there is a master plan. Look how little old me got to travel and study! I am still a student at age eighty-one. Longevity is not a thing for me. Quality is more important than quantity."

Ruth and Gerald, her husband of sixty-five years, helped found the Ben Eion ski hill in Cape Breton in 1968; Ruth was an instructor there in winters for fifty years.

Ruth passed away unexpectedly in 2018 at age eighty-two. The ski hill has since named the bunny hill Boutilier's Beginner Hill in her honour. Ruth has been inducted into the New Dawn Women's Gallery of Fame in Cape Breton.

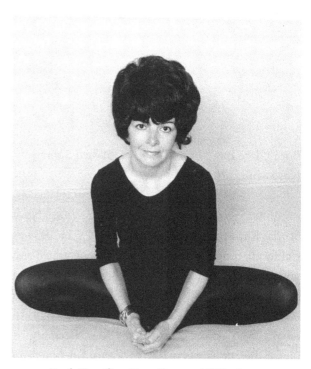

Ruth Boutilier, Cape Breton, 1975, photo Abbass Studio

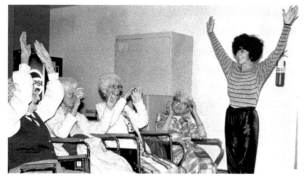

Ruth Boutilier teaching Seaview Nursing Home, Glace Bay, NS

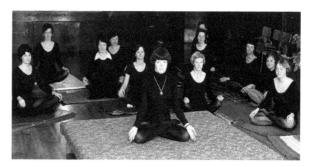

Ruth Boutilier teaching photo, Abbass Studio

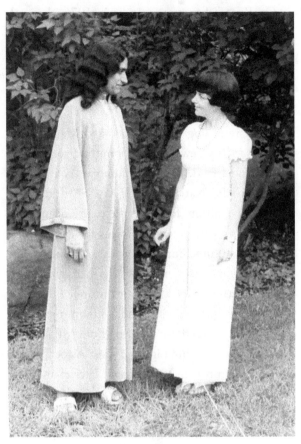

Amrit Desai and Ruth Boutilier, Reading,
Pennsyvlania, 1977

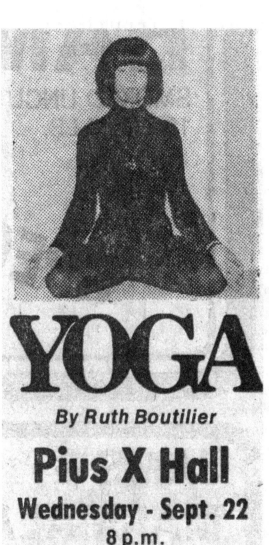

Ruth Boutilier, $5.00 class forever

Bruce Carruthers

Born Mahabaleshwar, India, 1933; died Vancouver, British Columbia, 2017

Bruce was notable as the first Canadian physician to recognize what therapeutic yoga could do to alleviate chronic symptoms, and for dedicating his life to advancing that cause.

Born and raised in India to missionary parents, he had a unique perspective of the Indian culture. His medical studies brought him to his father's alma mater in Kingston, Ontario, and eventually to Vancouver. Open to alternative health care, he was very receptive when his future wife, Maureen Tribe, introduced him to her newfound enthusiasm for Iyengar-style yoga.

Bruce was an internist with a special interest in myalgic encephalomyelitis (ME), more commonly known as chronic fatigue syndrome, and fibromyalgia (FM). He studied with BKS Iyengar in Pune, India, on several occasions. Together, with Mr. Iyengar's unique knowledge of the human body and the recuperative power of asana, a strong friendship formed between these two men. The friendship was built on a mutual desire to share knowledge that would help ease human suffering.

On Bruce's first trip to India in 1976, they collaborated on ways to spread Mr. Iyengar's groundbreaking new book, *Light on Pranayama,* to the west. An in-depth study of yogic classical breathing techniques, it was to become an indispensable teaching tool for westerners.

Upon returning home, Bruce and Maureen ran trainings at Thymeways, their home and yoga retreat on Galiano Island, British Columbia. As a medical advisor to the National ME/FM Network, Bruce gained recognition for his milestone advances in diagnostic and treatment protocols for these conditions. He lectured internationally and spent time with over 1,500 patients to study their symptoms, offer compassion, and share yoga for relief. He conducted workshops across Canada to train yoga teachers in ways to help those suffering from ME/FM.

Bruce founded the Light on Yoga Association in British Columbia in 1976, which later changed to the BKS Iyengar Association of Vancouver. It is still running today.

By the time Mr. Iyengar asked Bruce to spearhead his certification process in Canada in the 1990s, he verbally expressed skepticism about the certification process. He feared it would cause division rather than unity in the yoga community.

Bruce suffered a stroke in 2012 and thereafter lived at the Arbutus Care Centre in Vancouver, where he died in April 2017. Says one of his colleagues, Sherri Hunt-Todd: "Bruce was one of the most exceptional, interesting, and intuitive human beings I've ever met. I'm sure this played a great part in the legend he became to his friends, patients, colleagues, and throughout his many years of research. Patients really felt his compassion and respect for them."

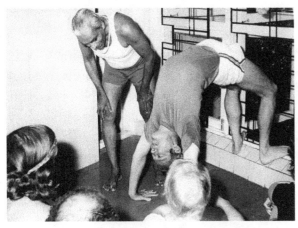

Bruce Carruthers being coached in backbend by
Mr. Iyengar

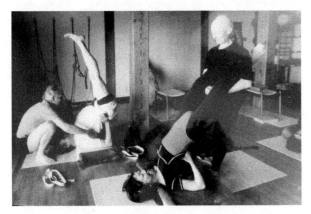

Maureen and Bruce Carruthers teaching
at Thymeways

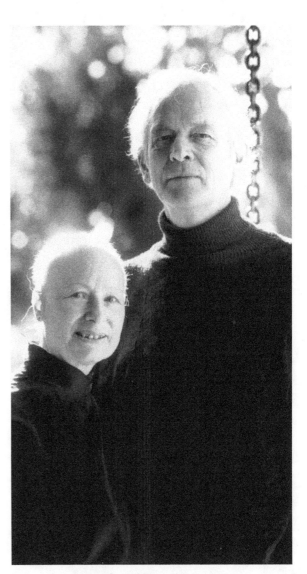

Maureen and Bruce Carruthers

Maureen Carruthers (Tribe)

Born Mana Park, England, 1939 –

Maureen is one of the first yoga teachers in the Vancouver area. She has spent a lifetime introducing people to yoga. In 1968, she began her first yoga classes with Jutta Wiedemann and later became a student of Bina Nelson's. Afflicted with dyslexia, she found that the practice of yoga helped her with concentration. She taught for several years in recreation centres in West Vancouver, and the Kerrisdale and Kitsilano areas, as well as for Langara College and the Vancouver School Board.

Maureen credits Donald Moyer of San Francisco for introducing her to the Iyengar style of yoga in 1974. She delved into Mr. Iyengar's book, *Light on Yoga,* and, along with her husband, physician Bruce Carruthers, arranged a trip to study with Mr. Iyengar at his institute in Pune, India. Bruce and Maureen shared a common purpose of wanting to make Iyengar yoga available in Canada to enhance the quality of people's lives.

In 1976 they held classes in their Kitsilano home, where Bruce also had his medical practice as an internist.

When they moved to Galiano Island in 1984 they created Thymeways, a retreat centre built into their home overlooking the Strait of Georgia. It was acclaimed as one of the first of its kind in Canada. On Mr. Iyengar's first trip to San Francisco (hosted by American Rama Vernon), he took a sidetrip to bless Thymeways at their grand opening. Students came from across Canada and the US to experience yoga in this idyllic setting. Maureen organized groups to take to the Iyengar institute in India, and many people credit their lifelong path in yoga to Maureen's generosity in assisting them to experience yoga in its motherland.

When Mr. Iyengar issued the first teaching certifications in Canada in 1997, he bestowed one each on Maureen and Bruce, as part of a group leading the Canadian certification process.

Although Maureen had reservations about the certification process, she remained faithful to this style. In a message to the next generation, she states: "I believe in a collective of people, not a hierarchy. A background in Iyengar yoga is wonderful, and then we need to move into our own genius. We need to trust our own instincts. I believe in apprenticeship, I believe in a collective where we all move as if from a large mandala to a unified centre. Do not be afraid to tread new ground, be who you are and be authentic, as Mr. Iyengar was."

Maureen trained and mentored many teachers who became successful in their own right, such as Norma Hodge, Susan Bull, and Ingelise Nherlan. Today, she is retired and an honorary member of the Iyengar Yoga Association of Canada.

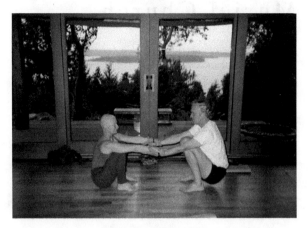

Bruce and Maureen Carruthers at home
Thymeways retreat

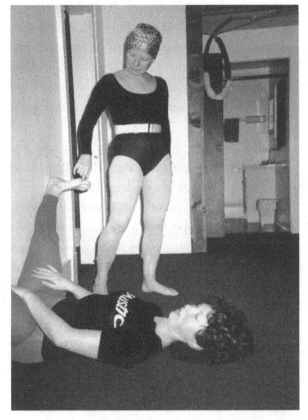

Maureen Carruthers in her home studio,
Vancouver 1980

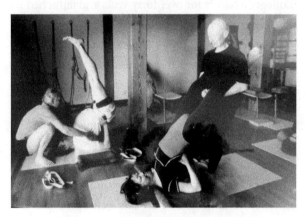

Maureen and Bruce Carruthers teaching
at Thymeways

Muriel Church

Born Toronto, Ontario, Canada, 1926; died Sarnia, Ontario, 2018

Muriel was the first in the Sarnia area to do a weekly yoga column in the local newspaper as well as a TV cable show. She taught yoga at Lambton College in Sarnia for over forty years and launched its first successful teacher training program, running it well into her late seventies. She taught at the YWCA, Fanshawe College, the Strangway Community Centre, and for the Collingwood ski team, all while finding time to serve on the board for Sarnia Hydro Commission. She was a founding member of the Federation of Ontario Yoga Teachers.

Her accomplishments were hard won.

Muriel contracted polio as a young girl and was confined to an iron bed for one year while she was recovering. This method was used in the 1930s and '40s to help keep patients' spines "straight," to lesson complications should paralysis occur. Polio left Muriel with some scoliosis, weakened lungs, and a weak right leg. Tough and determined, she started out on her road to recovery by becoming a competitive swimmer, but she had to give up due to breathing difficulties. A nun she knew recommended she take up yoga, which she did, and she experienced dramatic results. She taught herself from Kareen Zebroff's book, *The ABC of Yoga,* and later took trainings in Toronto. Inspired by Swami Rama of the Himalayan tradition and Swami Radha of the Sivananda tradition, she devoted herself to a three-year teacher training locally with Yogi Krishan Sidhu of Orillia, Ontario, where she received initiation as Swami Mehram Devi. Following the loss of her husband at a young age and one of her four daughters to breast cancer, Muriel's spiritual practice helped her through.

Muriel had a loyal following for years and was loved for her lively spirit and larger-than-life personality. She encouraged her students to start the day off by drinking hot water with honey and lemon, followed by single-pointed focus meditation. She was famous for her trademark yoga gym suits and her chic hats. She owned hundreds of hats and was seldom seen without one.

Student Jennifer Adam interviewed Muriel for *Yoga International* magazine in 2017. "Meet Muriel, my ninety-year-old yoga teacher," she wrote. Said Muriel from her nursing home: "I am in my ninetieth year and currently in a controlled environment. Without yoga, I would not have had the positive attitude and the mental and physical skills required to continue on with life, given my polio and post-polio syndrome, and now my loss of independence. It is the philosophy and the science of yoga that have helped me continue to see a purpose in my life beyond my physical ability. I truly believe that

I would not have lived so long and so well without yoga—and, of course, my wonderful family."

Muriel was teaching about a dozen faithful seniors from her wheelchair until she died at age ninety-one, but not before she happily gave away all her treasured hats and yoga books. She gave her original copy of *The ABC of Yoga* by Kareen Zebroff to a friend of her grandson, who, coincidentally, opened a yoga studio in Kareen's birthplace of Germany.

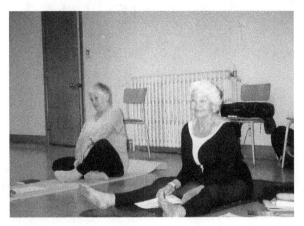

Muriel Church (right) at age 80

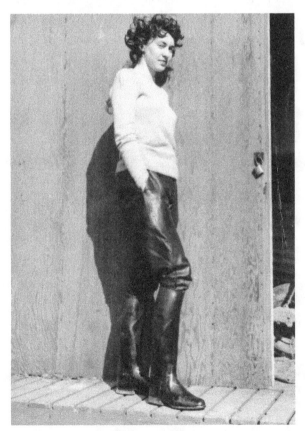

Young Muriel Church

Bishwambhar Dass

Born Winnipeg, Manitoba, Canada, 1948 –

Bishwambhar Dass had a specific dream of meeting an Indian mystic teacher as a young boy. Many years later he read the book known as the counter-culture bible of the time, *Be Here Now,* by Ram Dass, a former Harvard psychology professor who became famous for going to India and studying with a mystic named Baba Hari Dass. So, when Bishwambhar saw a poster at the Fifth Kingdom bookstore in Toronto advertising an upcoming workshop with Baba Hari Dass in Vancouver, he was determined to meet him. He hitchhiked across the country and had a private meeting with him. He experienced the "shock of recognition" that so often happens when an erstwhile student meets their authentic guru. He remembered his vivid dream from when he was a child. Thus began Bishwambhar's life-long relationship with Baba Hari Dass.

Baba Hari Dass was known as the "silent monk" after taking a vow of silence in India in 1952; he nevertheless was able to pierce to the heart of anyone's questions by writing a succinct answer on a small chalkboard that he carried on a string around his neck. He drew from the philosophy of Patanjali's eight limbs (Ashtanga Yoga) and the sacred text of the *Bhagavad Gita* in his teachings.

Bishwambhar Dass was given his name by Baba Hari Dass, who initiated him based partially on his astrological chart. Bishwambhar means "supreme spirit" and *Dass* means "servant of God." Bishwambhar returned to Toronto where a circle of devotees formed, including Andrea Roth (Lakshmi) and Alan Trimble (Anand Dass). They formed a group to teach Ashtanga Yoga philosophy that matched the dedication of the West Coast devotees, who were in the process of buying land to establish the Salt Spring Yoga Centre.

Bishwambhar and Alan founded the non-profit Ashtanga Yoga Fellowship (AYF) in 1976. Along with Andrea, they became successful yoga teachers in their own right and gave birth to a project that was to have an influence in Canada for the next thirty-seven years. Ashtanga Yoga Fellowship (later to be called Yogastock, Inc.) offered summer yoga camps, attracting up to 150 people each year on properties outside of Aurora, Ontario. They brought in tents and cooking facilities, set up stages for kirtan concerts and nets for volleyball. The daily schedule resembled that of an Indian-style ashram, with a disciplined practice before breakfast at eleven, including *arati* (morning prayer of light), chanting, bodily purifications such as neti pots and tongue cleansers (*shatkarma*), pranayama, and meditation. Study classes included the *Bhagavad Gita* or the *Yoga Sutras* and evenings were satsang (evening fellowship) and kirtan.

The children attending these camps often quote the memorable playtime they had with Baba Hari Dass, describing him as loving, fun, and mischievous. The evening gatherings were full of infectious laughter. His gentle, childlike nature endeared him to all and was a contrast to his keen intellectual mind, which took on the most profound riddles of the universe.

By featuring Baba Hari Dass and his teachings through the family camps, AYF shaped the minds of the future. Jessica Robertson, who often attended with her parents as a young girl, went on to found the famous international Moda (formerly Moksha) yoga studio chain, infusing tenets of the eight limbs of yoga such as *aparigraha* (non-hoarding) and *ahimsa* (non-violence) as part of her company's mission statement. Bishwambhar's son, Josh McKay, grew up to complete a thesis at the University of British Columbia on the effects of yogic breathing (*pranayama*) on the human body. Countless people have written to thank AYF for teaching them valuable life skills that positively influenced them and their children, continuing the generational imprint of peaceful living and selfless service.

Bishwambar, Alan, and Andrea Roth-Trimble all live in the Queensville, Ontario area where they continue to teach and sustain a yoga community. Yogastock Inc.'s thirty-eighth annual summer camp was cancelled due to lack of numbers, giving these senior teachers time to reflect on the many blessings received through Baba Hari Dass and perhaps hear his next words to them. Baba Hari Dass passed away at his home at Mount Madonna Center in California on September 25, 2018, at the age of ninety-five.

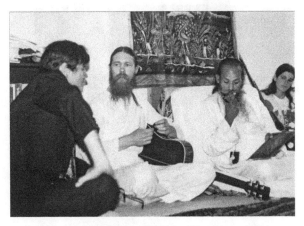

Bishwambhar Dass with Baba Hari Dass, 1974

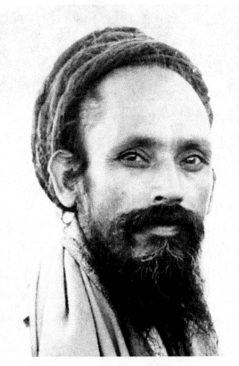

Baba Hari Dass

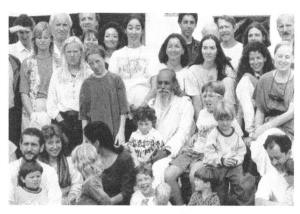

Yogastock summer retreat

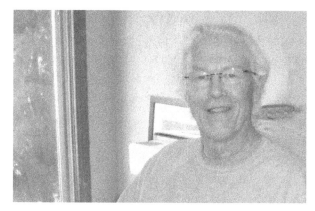

Bishwambhar Dass today

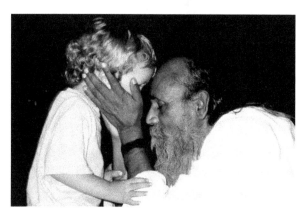

Baba Hari and Josh McKay age four

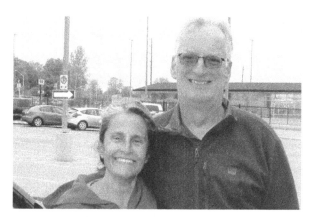

Andrea and Alan Trimble Yogastock

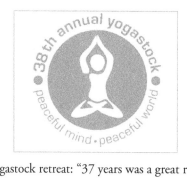

Yogastock retreat: "37 years was a great run"

Lone Eriksen-Parker

Born Ubby, Denmark, 1946 –

Lone (pronounced Lonah) immigrated to Canada in 1966. She immediately found Richard Hittleman's book, *Yoga: 28 Day Exercise Plan,* and started practicing. She followed with Paramahansa Yogananda's *Autobiography of a Yogi,* published by the Self Realization Fellowship (SRF), and took training with SRF in meditation and kriya techniques. She liked the heartfelt approach and became initiated in that tradition at SRF Los Angeles in 1980. During the process, she taught everything she knew to others, and became one of the first teachers in New Brunswick. Later, she became certified in the Kripalu style of yoga.

In her desire to help others, she became a social worker in 1991 through St. Thomas University in Fredericton, New Brunswick. She applied the principles of yoga therapy to her clients in the mental health field as well as to her coworkers, helping establish yoga as a recognized healing modality. Her work included teaching postures, breath work, and visualization and relaxation techniques.

As a social worker, first in child protection services and then private practice, her yoga skills became more in demand. She set up formal classes at the University of New Brunswick, high schools, government departments, and mental health clinics.

And then life threw her a curve ball. Lone was in a car accident and suffered a broken pelvis that left her flat on her back for a month in the hospital. She was sixty years old. This is when everything she knew about yoga and recovery kicked in—there was no time for self-pity. She used her knowledge of *pranayama* (yogic breathing) and visualization faithfully. "My first insight was that I had been given precious time and there was an opportunity here for practice at a deeper, more subtle level," she recalls. "Rather than resist the experience, I embraced it as the student I've always been. I was powerless over the injury but I had powerful tools to recover." When she resumed teaching a year later, she found herself even better equipped to guide others in recovery.

Lone currently sees several clients a week through her work with Health Canada. Some of these clients are from the nearby Gagetown military base and some suffer from PTSD. Says Lone: "They are locked in fear and I teach them how to breathe, relax, watch, and feel. I show them how emotions are triggered by thoughts and memories. If we have compassion for these thoughts and memories when they come up, they can be valuable teachers." Through her company, Life Balance Through Yoga, she conducts seminars on Remember Your Sacred Self and life balance, teaching people her specific yoga techniques. Says Lone: "A crisis is an invitation to wake up to the present moment, embrace the now, and to use the contents in our lives to set us free—to go beyond the dualities of pleasure and pain and to let go of attachments and aversion. A health crisis that results in the loss of body function can help us deeply understand who we are beyond the body. The crisis is an invitation to go within."

When asked about the solitary journey of teaching in New Brunswick, Lone says, "It wasn't hard for me to pioneer yoga. It is a force inside that drives me. I really didn't do anything but follow it. My practice gives me great inner peace and roots me in ME. My license plate of twenty-two years spells PEACE. When some people remark that world peace is impossible, I remind them. I am talking about a rich inner peace accessible to us all, and it begins with you."

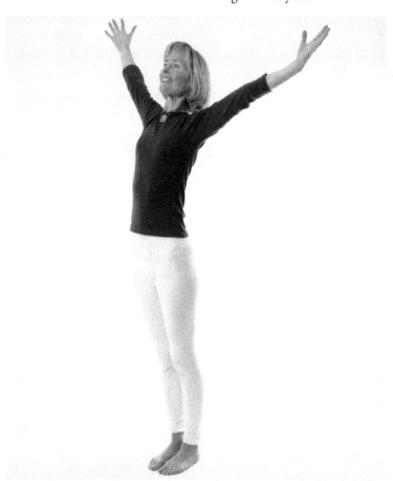

Lone Eriksen-Parker, Fredericton, New Brunswick

Shirley Daventry French

Born London, England, 1931 –

There is a charming yoga centre on Fort Street in Victoria that is worth a visit. It has been through many changes since its inception and there are many contributors to its success. However, it would not have happened without the vision and dedication of its founder, Shirley Daventry French.

Shirley took her first yoga class at the Victoria YWCA with Jessica Tucker in 1970. Yoga classes were considered edgy at the time, but Shirley was seeking. When Jessica invited Swami Radha of the Yasodhara Ashram in Kootenay Bay, British Columbia to give a series of talks on yoga philosophy, Shirley attended and felt an instant rapport with her teachings. She began annual summer visits to the ashram, along with her physician husband, Derek French, and graduated from the three-month residential Yasodhara Teacher Training Program in 1976. It was there, while taking Iyengar classes with Norma Hodge, that she deepened her appreciation of the Iyengar style of yoga and delved into his book *Light on Yoga.*

Encouraged by Swami Radha to create a space for *satsang* (fellowship), Shirley, along with founding members Carol Miller, Donna Fornelli, and her husband, Derek, created the Yoga Centre of Victoria in 1977. It was formed as a non-profit society with a board of directors, and remains so to this day. The centre brought teachers in to help advance their skills—Americans like Ramanand Patel and Donald Moyer played a prominent role by teaching workshops, followed by Maureen and Bruce Carruthers, Angela Farmer, and many others. Shirley visited and trained with Mr. Iyengar at his institute in Pune, India, a total of fifteen times over her lifetime. Her husband, also an avid practitioner, and, as close friends of Mr. Iyengar, they advocated for his work in Canada. In 1997, along with ten others, she was part of the first tier who received Iyengar certification in Canada.

When asked about her accomplishments, Shirley responds, "I am happy I was able to be of service to Mr. Iyengar and earn his trust as a writer, editor, and teacher of his method of yoga. I was honoured to establish a centre for this work in Victoria, mentor many of Canada's senior teachers, and establish a well-regarded newsletter. I feel rewarded that I am now in a position that this work has gained its own momentum and no longer needs me." Shirley is the editor of the biography, *Iyengar: His Life and Work*, and one of the editors of Mr. Iyengar's *Light on the Yoga Sutras of Patanjali.* Shirley stepped down from the board of directors of the Yoga Centre of Victoria (now called the Iyengar Yoga Centre of Victoria) in

2011, but continues to serve on their teacher training committee.

Shirley's advice to the next generation of yogis is her favorite quote from Swami Vivekananda: "Discard everything that weakens you."

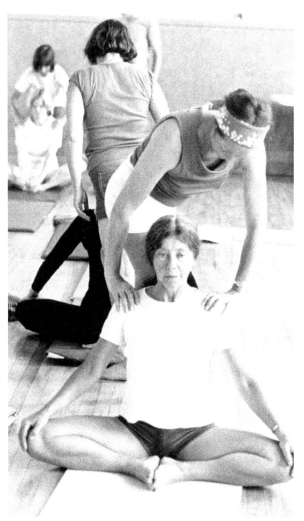

Shirley Daventry French

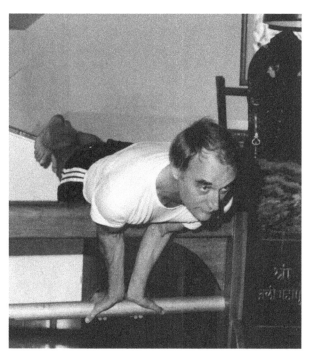

Derek French doing Chataranga, Iyengar Institute.

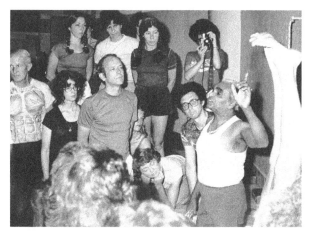

Shirley French (centre) Iyengar Institute, 1979

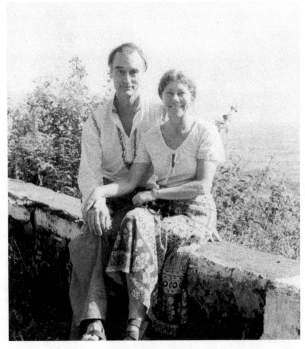

Shirley and Derek French

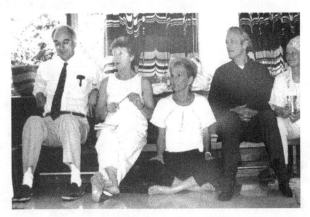

Derek and Shirley French, Liz McLeod,
Bruce and Maureen Carruthers

Lloyd Kreitzer

Born Valdosta, Georgia, United States, 1944 –

Lloyd's first exposure to yoga was in 1956 in southern California where he grew up—his aunt did a yoga demo at her Christmas party when he was twelve years old. He was encouraged to try it and when he went instantly into lotus pose, his aunt declared, "That is a gift. Don't lose it!" Those words were to resonate in him well into the future—many years later, he would become the first yoga teacher in a little-known place called Regina, Saskatchewan.

Lloyd spent two years as a Peace Corps volunteer in Malaysian Borneo, where he ignited a lifelong love of plants while studying tropical agriculture. Years later, he would have occasion to use this knowledge while taking care of fruit tree orchards at Swami Radha's Yasodhara Ashram in Kootenay Bay, British Columbia.

Once home in the US, Lloyd experienced a culture shock that spurred deep inquiry. He showed up for a yoga class after seeing an ad and began to practice in earnest. He made it his personal motive that year of 1970 to learn self-discipline through yoga. "I was ripe and ready and focused and I was a

zealot," says Lloyd. In 1971, he studied with Swami Vishnudevananda for one year in New York City.

In September 1972, he fell in love and followed his sweetheart to her home in Saskatchewan. Once in Regina, he saw a poster advertising yoga classes at the University of Regina. Noting with interest that the instructor shared the same Sivananda training, he phoned the university to inquire. They informed him that the instructor was an American and, unfortunately, had just been called home to his family. They went further to say they were stranded with two fully registered classes and no teacher. Would Lloyd like to teach them? The answer was an emphatic yes!

In no time at all he was teaching up to seventeen classes a week all over the city. When he taught in a room above an ice hockey rink, the students asked how they were supposed to concentrate with all that noise. Lloyd replied, "The purpose of the practice is to develop concentration, no matter where you are."

Lloyd thrived in his job. "It is such a privilege. There is no higher calling than teaching yoga. Practice helps each of us express the gratitude of waking up consciously," he says "There is no difference between yoga styles. It's about returning to the Self and allowing the Self to be creative. I was so grateful to be teaching."

To him, the value was not in his students seeing him as a teacher, but in helping them see their own teacher within—he took it as a personal challenge to practice detachment from the power of being a teacher.

"There should be a twelve-step program for the addiction of teaching. The Buddhist teaching of non-attachment says you can become too connected to your identity as a teacher. So it is another practice to be detached from your attachment to teaching!

"I wanted my students to have the same intense commitment that I had. I never lost an opportunity to teach them that discipline brought rewards. We wake up to the brilliance of being human beings with a vast capacity to love."

After returning to the US, Lloyd settled in Albuquerque, New Mexico, where he runs an organic nursery and works as a nature therapy guide, drawing from his years of studying yoga. "I teach people how to deepen connection in all that they do by approaching each task as a communion with the Divine, extracting the richness of each moment and sharing it generously with others."

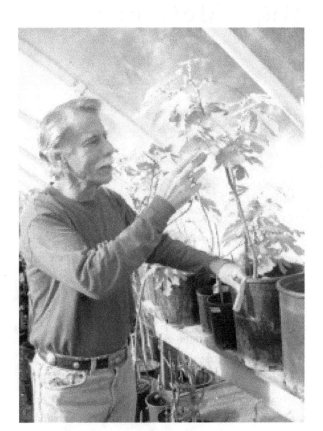

Lloyd Kreitzer, 2018 Albuquerque, New Mexico

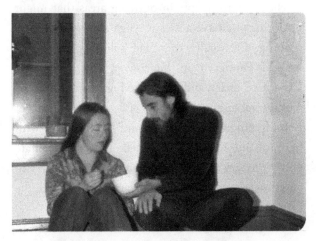

Gloria Saur and Lloyd Kreitzer, Regina,
Saskatchewan, 1972

Mugs McConnell

Born Creston, British Columbia, Canada, 1955 –

Marion McConnell, affectionately called "Mugs," is one of Canada's earliest yoga ambassadors. She is the first Canadian representative for the International Yoga Teachers Association (IYTA), headed in Sydney, Australia, co-founder of the South Okanagan Yoga Association (SOYA), and the only recipient of the Queen Elizabeth II Diamond Jubilee Award for promoting yoga in Canada and abroad.

Mugs was first introduced to yoga when she was seventeen. "My neighbour introduced me to Transcendental Meditation ® and I wanted to learn yoga, too. She invited me over to practice on TV with Kareen Zebroff and I went out and bought her book, *The ABC of Yoga*."

In 1974, Mugs moved to Australia, where she found yoga classes and became acquainted with the IYTA, beginning a lifelong association. She also discovered Dr. Hari Dickman, a Latvian yogi living in California who started the Latvian Yoga Society in the 1930s and who taught yoga in displaced persons camps during and after World War II. He was distinguished for having studied with many acknowledged masters, and once released from the camps he left Europe to be close to his personal teacher, the famous Paramahansa Yogananada. Yogananda died only two months after Dr. Dickman arrived in the US in 1952, and prior to their having met.

When Mugs moved to Santa Cruz, California, as a serious student, Dr. Dickman tutored her in the deeper philosophies and practices of yoga. At his urging, she lived at various Sivananda ashrams worldwide and attended the first teacher training at the Sivananda Ashram in the Bahamas with Swami Vishnudevananda, graduating in 1978. She completely absorbed and breathed the Sivananda style. She returned to Dr. Dickman's home as a student, where she remained until he died in 1979.

Mugs moved home and taught in Penticton and area for over thirty years. She co-founded SOYA in 1995 with fellow teacher Dariel Vogel. Likening themselves to a tree with many branches, SOYA reached out to people in outlying areas that might not otherwise have access to yoga and yoga teacher training. Eventually they had solid representation beyond Penticton in Vancouver, Prince George, Creston, Calgary, and Mexico. Mugs teaches or oversees several annual 200- and 300-hour yoga teacher training programs in Canada and Mexico along with her husband, Robert McConnell. They also facilitate yearly retreats in the Okanagan, bringing over 120 yogis together to learn from greats from Canada, the US, and India.

Mugs is one of the few Canadians to study in depth the intricacies of yoga mantras and pujas, becoming certified by American expert Namadeva

Acharya (Thomas Ashley Farrand, 1940-2010). She has presented several times at the international conferences of the IYTA. Says Mugs: "I spoke from personal experience. In 1984 in Barcelona, I spoke on yoga and backpacking: using yoga techniques to survive the wilderness. I shared what I had learned from practicing the eight limbs of yoga while backpacking the Pacific Crest Trail in 1979 and also on the Continental Divide in 1983. My sister and I covered over 5,000 miles trekking in the wilderness while practicing mental yoga! I also presented at the 1997 congress on Karma and Reincarnation: Using the Yamas and Niyamas to Overcome the Five Obstacles. I was really into it!"

Mugs is on the board of directors of Yoga Alliance, a US-based yoga school and teacher registry, and has served on several YA committees over the years.

She is author of *Letters from the Yoga Masters*, a book of notable inspirational and instructional letters from the great masters of late nineteenth and early twentieth century India, written to her teacher Dr. Dickman back in the war and postwar days.

After many years living in British Columbia and Mexico, Mugs and Robert relocated to a new home near Waterton Lakes National Park, Alberta, in the foothills of the Rockies. From here, she travels and teaches yoga workshops based on her lifelong studies.

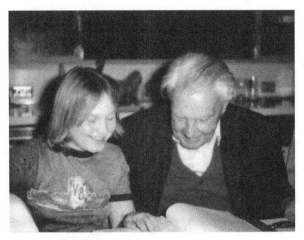

Young Mugs McConnell with Dr. Hari Dickman 1975

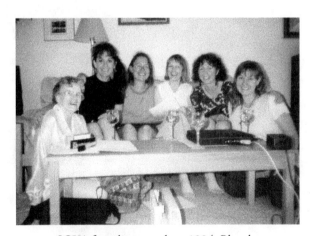

SOYA founding members 1994: Blanche Livingston, Dariel Vogel, Meui McKiblin, Mugs McConnell, Marsha Saldat, Michele Kuhla

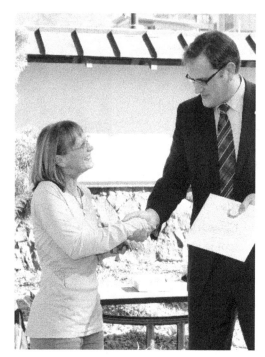

Mugs receiving Queens Diamond Jubilee Award

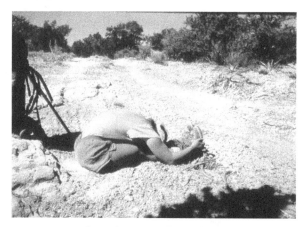

Hiking Continental Divide Trail

Lois Morrison

Born Saskatoon, Saskatchewan, 1932 –

Lois is the first known yoga teacher in Saskatoon, starting in 1971.

Lois earned a physical education degree from the University of Saskatoon and had a genuine love of fitness. In yoga, she started off with Richard Hittleman's and Kareen Zebroff's books and Kareen's TV series. Except for a weekend workshop she took in Calgary, Lois was entirely self-taught. By her third year of teaching, she was teaching beginner, intermediate, and advanced classes. She started teaching at the YWCA, where she stayed for the next thirty-five years, followed by classes for men at the downtown Saskatoon YMCA. "Their wives brought them, but they did get there," chuckles Lois. For a while, Lois taught aerobics and fitness classes interspersed with yoga, but when people kept asking for relaxation at the end of the class, she decided to focus on yoga and meditation.

Lois was involved with Girl Guides of Canada for over seventy-two years. She has been a guest teacher, introducing yoga and meditation to Girl Guides for some thirty-five years. For her contribution to GGC, she has received the Beaver Badge, their highest award in Canada. For a time, Lois also worked part time as a provincial commissioner for Saskatoon in a volunteer advisory role, training people in the prevention of child abuse.

Lois bridges her Christian faith with yoga. She has been a member of her parents' church, Christ Church Anglican, her entire life and serves on the vestry today, lending creative ideas and hard work to help save the church in stressful financial times.

Because Lois's husband's travelled a great deal with his job, Lois had reliable childcare in the evenings for many years, allowing her to teach yoga in rural areas. She set up registered classes in many small towns surrounding Saskatoon and drove across the prairies in the most severe winter conditions to introduce people to yoga.

Lois taught at community centres and seniors' complexes, as well as classes for plus-size ladies above the dress shop in downtown Saskatoon. She remembers a funny story from when she taught a night class in a pharmacy. Everyone was on the floor in the dark in *savasana*—final relaxation translated as "corpse" pose—when a policeman walked by and saw them through the window. Thinking it was a robbery, he frantically started trying to knock the door down!

Lois has lost her husband, but is still going strong at eighty-seven years young. She teaches five classes a week at the Cosmo Seniors Centre, and remains a living icon of yoga in Saskatoon.

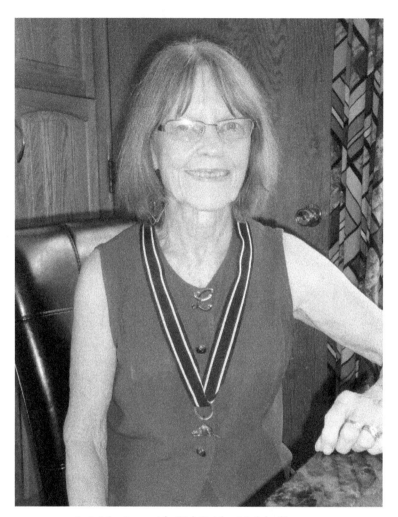

Lois Morrison with Girl Guides Medal of honour

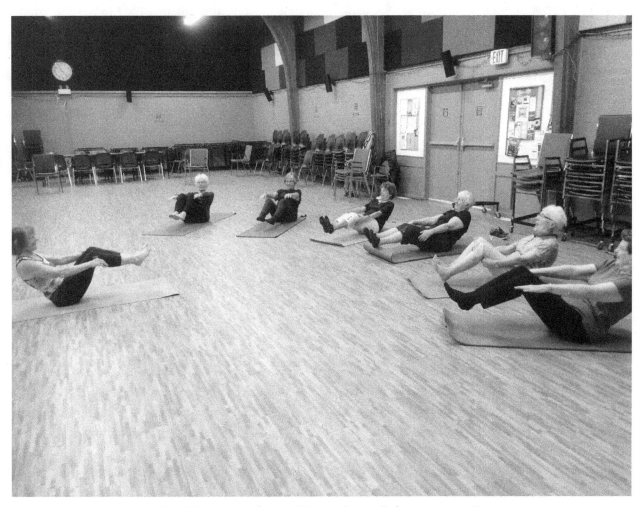

Lois Morrison teaching at Cosmos Centre, Saskatoon, at age 87

Bina Nelson

Born Allahabad, India,1918; died Vancouver, British Columbia, 1992

Bina Nelson was a woman of distinction. She is credited with setting up some of the first yoga programs in both eastern and western Canada in the 1960s. She also opened the first yoga studio in Vancouver and the Lower Mainland of British Columbia

Adventurous, business savvy, and determined, Bina was way ahead of her time. She was affectionately called "the Bengali tiger" by her students because of her firm teaching style and fierce dedication to her art. She wore her trademark sari while teaching, and students looked forward to the half-hour relaxation at the beginning of each class.

Originally from Allahabad, India, Bina was encouraged in yoga by her Methodist minister father, who was a yoga practitioner. Bina was destined to be a leader—she travelled alone, even though it was unusual for a woman to do so in the 1940s and '50s. Her adventurous streak took her to study first in Calcutta and then to Washington State College, where she earned a master of science degree, then to New York University, where she became the first Indian woman to obtain a PhD in physical education. She returned briefly to Calcutta, where she worked at the YWCA, then returned to the US as an exchange PE professor in Hampton, Virginia.

By the time she made Canada her home, she had a reputation as a yoga expert. She stayed briefly in Halifax, Nova Scotia, where she set up yoga programs at the YWCA in the mid-1960s. She travelled throughout the Maritimes, lecturing and introducing people to yoga at a time when yoga was mostly unknown.

Bina moved to Vancouver in 1966 to be with her brother, Delip Nelson. She set up a company called Yoga Fitness in 1968 and took her business cards around, enthusiastically knocking on doors and offering to speak to, teach, or otherwise inspire people about yoga. She sold colleges on the merits of including yoga in their physical education programs.

Simon Fraser University agreed to test Bina's vision and launched yoga programs, as did the YWCA on Burrard Street. They flourish to this day.

As a yoga businesswoman long before it was deemed acceptable, Bina lifted yoga out of church basements and into a professional setting. She opened Vancouver's first yoga studio, called the Yoga Fitness Institute, on West Broadway in Kitsilano in 1970. As shrewd as she was adventurous, she later bought the building.

Bina loved to draw people around her, offering Indian cooking classes and meditation gatherings and successfully establishing a yoga community.

Bina never married nor had children. She considered herself first and foremost an ambassador of yoga. As a pioneer and a foreigner, she broke down barriers in Canada to make her dream come true. She set up the first teacher training program in Vancouver and often took her trainees with her to give demonstrations at seniors' centres, youth programs, churches, and institutions. Bina passed away in 1992, but her legacy lives on through the teachers she has trained.

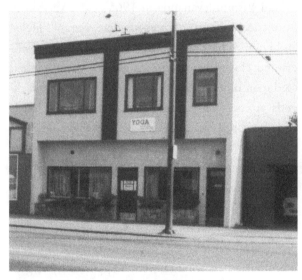

Yoga Fitness Institute, Broadway Ave.
Vancouver, 1968

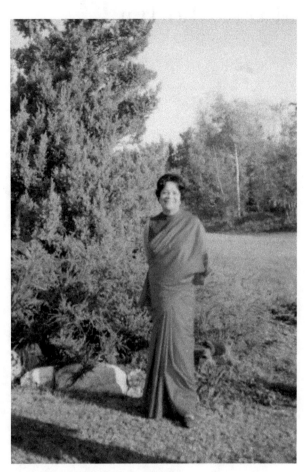

Bina Nelson teacher, educator, entrepreneur

Marie Paulyn

Born Bayonne, France, 1927; died Toronto,
Ontario, 2017

Marie was born and raised in France, studied
philosophy and religion at Sorbonne University, and
eventually immigrated to Montreal in the 1940s
with her family.

Later, when she moved to Toronto, she was an
actress with a French theatre group. A modelling and
acting career included early television commercials
for coffee, soaps, and even cigarettes, although this
was something she laughed about later in life.

Her great-grandmother, who was a follower of
the famous occultist Madame Blavatsky, influenced
Marie's father toward the supernatural. One day in
the kitchen, he told her about the great mystical yogis
of India. She recalls that moment vividly: "Standing
there listening to his words, I felt this deep feeling
grip me. I made my mind up right there and then
that I would go to India one day."

Eventually, Marie was to fulfill her childhood
pledge. She went to Rishikesh, India, to meet the
gurus firsthand, and studied internationally with
some prominent teachers.

First, life took its course. Marie got married and
had children. But her marriage was faltering and
her career travelling globally doing trade shows for
a Toronto fashion company was stressful—and she
was a chronic insomniac. With her father's words
still resonating in her, she took up yoga and threw
away her sleeping pills. She started classes with
John and Tinie Gollop, the first yoga studio owners
in Ontario. She then obtained certification from
Swami Vishnudevananda in 1965 at the Val Morin
Sivananda Ashram in Quebec. Here, she met Helen
and Franz Achatz of Toronto, who became her teachers and close friends. She taught for them at their
studio on Bloor Street in 1971, and later spent weekends at their retreat in Eganville, Ontario. Marie
simultaneously maintained her lifelong studies in
mysticism and philosophy, becoming a member
of the Association of Humanistic Psychology and
studying at the University of Toronto.

In 1975, Marie was a founding member of
Federation of Ontario Yoga Teachers, FOYT, a non-
profit group promoting yoga provincially. She was
keen that others would have the opportunity to gain
the richness of yoga philosophy that she had received.
She dedicated twenty-five years of her life to this
effort through FOYT by teaching workshops and
trainings, and also served on their executive board.

Marie liked to tell the story of how she opened
her first yoga studio in 1972. While applying for a
government job, the last question on the interview
form was, "What is your hobby?" When she wrote
"yoga" they asked her to change her answer because

that they did not want to be linked to "that weird practice." They gave her forty-eight hours to give it up and sign the contract. She went home and made a spiritual plea in her meditation. She decided that if she found a yoga space within forty-eight hours that could fit twenty people, she would open a school. The next morning, she was on Yonge Street and saw an office for rent. It was 1,000 square feet and cost $300 a month. Needless to say, she called her would-be employer with an emphatic "No" in answer to their request.

She had a vibrant studio, the Hatha and Raja Yoga School, for eleven years. The teachers in training would meet one night a week and cover one asana (pose) per evening in depth.

When the building was sold, she taught out of her house. Although her home was a haven of warmth for many, it eventually became too small. So in 2004, her students arranged for her to teach at the Royal Canadian Yacht Club, the Granite Club, and Simon Church. She taught there until her diagnosis of cancer at the age of eighty-nine.

At the time off her passing, Marie had three children, four grandchildren, and three great-grandchildren; she had trained 250 teachers and had thousands of grateful students. She had a spiritual radiance that drew people to her.

Her favourite quote about yoga to newcomers was, "Keep practicing! Four thousand years of satisfied customers can't be wrong!"

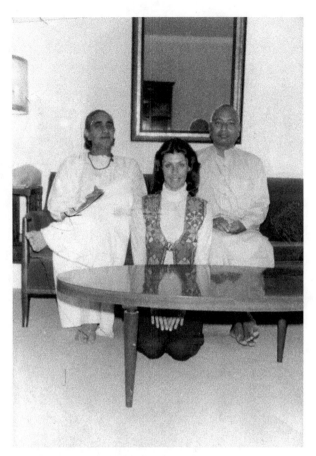

Swami Rama, Marie Paulyn, Swami Venkatesananda, 1974

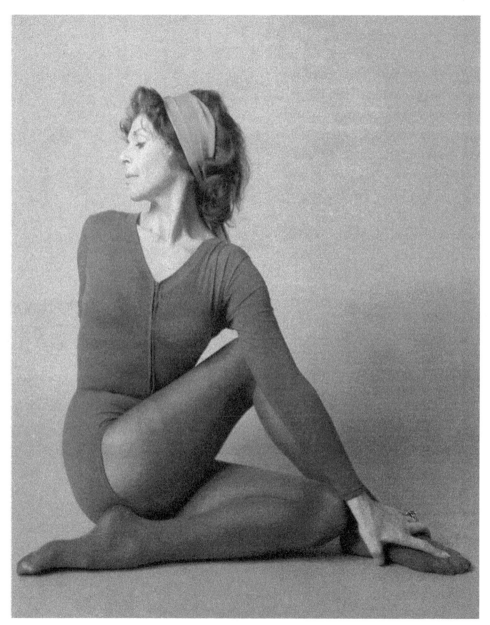

Marie Paulyn, *Homemakers* magazine, 1975

Hilda Pezarro

Born Wintook, South Africa, 1931; died Vancouver, British Columbia, 2017

Hilda's curious mind about mysticism and spirituality was always prevalent. So when she accompanied her husband, Leo, with his geophysical work in the UK and Pakistan, she explored various disciplines, including yoga while in Australia. When they eventually settled in Edmonton, Canada, she became a teacher from Friedel Khattab's School of Yoga's first graduating class in 1970.

Hilda became Calgary's first known yoga teacher, followed by Bonnie Dunbar. Her classes at the Jubilee Auditorium Theatre and Cultural Centre were always full.

In the 1970s, she began studying with Swami Radha at the Yasodhara Ashram in Kootenay Bay, British Columbia. She developed a close relationship with the swami, referring to her as "the mother I never had." After being introduced to the Iyengar style of yoga through Norma Hodge at the ashram, she travelled to Pune, India to train with Mr. Iyengar personally. Seeking even more depth to her spiritual practice, she also studied Buddhist philosophy.

Hilda was ahead of her time in teaching yoga and meditation and trying out health food fads, and people were drawn to her progressive personality. It drew a few chuckles when her husband was asked to speak at the Yoga Association of Alberta's annual meeting in 1996. "I've worked all over the world and I am the president of an oil company, but whenever I am introduced people say, 'Oh, aren't you the guy married to that yoga lady?'"

Hilda gave years of service to the executive board of the Yoga Association of Alberta in its formative years in the 1970s and '80s, establishing programs to fill the hunger for yoga in the rural areas and helping set up teacher training standards. She was also a founding member of the Iyengar Yoga Association of Canada.

Hilda died in October 2017, of dementia. In her early stages of the disease, she used her meditation and life philosophy admirably to help cope. She is survived by four children; Chris and Mark are Iyengar yoga teachers.

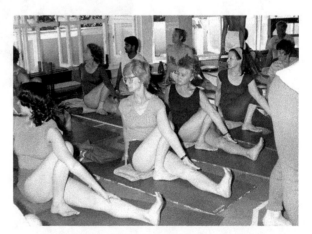

Hilda Pezarro (centre, glasses), Calgary's first yoga teacher

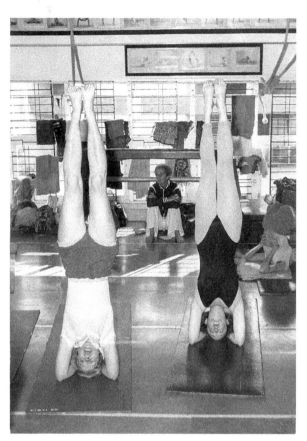

Hilda Pezarro (left) in headstand, Liz McLeod (centre) person right unknown

Sandra Sammartino

Born Trail, British Columbia, 1941 –

Sandra is referred to by some as the "grandmother of yoga." Known for being an unconventional and heartfelt pioneer and educator, she is responsible for much of today's West Coast yoga scene.

Young Sandra attended the University of British Columbia and became an elementary school teacher, followed by marriage and three children. When her marriage broke down at age twenty-nine, Sandra had what she calls a '"nervous breakdown," though she was later to describe it as a "breakthrough." Sandra says: "I was prescribed valium and I cried a lot. I didn't know what the next step was."

Her mother had done yoga with Kareen Zebroff and recommended Sandra give it a try. In 1971, she joined classes with Deedee Poyner at Vancouver's second studio, the Vancouver Yoga Centre. She immediately felt benefit. Around the same, time she signed up for a university course called Voluntary Control of Internal States with meditation teacher Jack Schwartz. Sandra credits her training with Schwartz for helping her understand her *kundalini* energy system and its awakening at a time when she was in psychological and emotional turmoil. She learned to develop it and use

its intuitive guidance. She remained Schwartz's student for the next fifteen years. She gained confidence as she learned how to draw from her spiritual source and she grew in popularity as a teacher.

Sandra was introduced to Iyengar yoga through Maureen Tribe (later to become Maureen Carruthers), who was teaching in Kitsilano in Vancouver at the time. She liked the challenge of this new style on the scene and committed to it entirely. She accompanied Maureen and her group on a 1977 trip to India to study with Mr. Iyengar.

Sandra received her Iyengar certification, but states, "I was kicked out of the association for not following their rules." She surrendered her certification when they requested, and trusted in herself going forward, as her training with Jack Schwartz had taught her to do.

Sandra accepted the support of forward thinker Rama Vernon of Seattle in her next steps. Rama was a visionary and a powerful driving force behind organizing yoga in the US. Living in Seattle, Rama was close enough to help Sandra launch her first teacher training program in 1980. It was a hugely successful program, held first in Vancouver, and later at Sandra's new yoga centre, Kairos, in White Rock. Sandra's program ran for the next fifteen years, and it launched many successful teachers into the second generation of yoga.

Sandra did TV shows on community cable television. Then, inspired by Anabelle Tame of the UK's Phoenix Rising Prison program, Sandra founded Yoga Outreach in 1992, a non-profit organization offering yoga to those without access. The program is still running today, serving prisons, women's centres, youth facilities, and transition houses.

Sandra lives in White Rock, British Columbia, with her husband, Bob. She has five children and six grandchildren, as well as her extensive yoga family. She conducts workshops locally and retreats at Kingfisher Lodge on Vancouver Island. She has made it a personal mission to increase awareness of the headstand and shoulder stand practice, which she calls the king and queen of asana. She states, "The practice of these two important poses give lots of health benefits and youthfulness and vibrancy. Sadly, they are overlooked by many current teachers today."

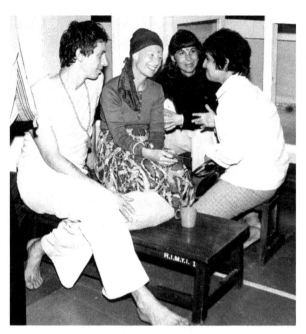

Maureen Carruthers and Sandra Sammartino (centre) with friends, Pune, India, 1979

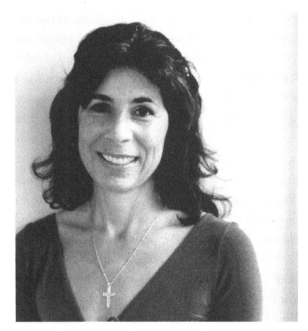

Young Sandra Sammartino, White Rock, British Columbia

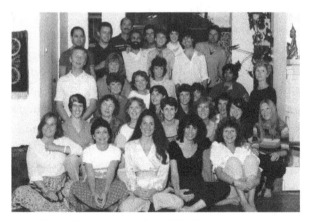

Rama Vernon (centre) and Sandra Sammartino (centre right) with first teacher training graduates, 1980

Bonnie Skinner

Born Regina, Saskatchewan, 1942 –

Bonnie Skinner started yoga on TV with Kareen Zebroff in the early 1970s and found it helped her chronic back pain. While living in Edmonton for a few years, she took Friedel Khattab's teacher training program in 1973. People were to remark later in her life that they knew she was a Khattab graduate due to her precise, no-nonsense approach. Bonnie began teaching in her basement, to one person! She looks back at those days incredulously.

Bonnie moved to Saskatchewan and started teaching yoga at the University of Regina, where she stayed for the next thirty-five years. Says Bonnie: "The rewards of being a teacher all these years have been immeasurable. I worked full time as an assistant to the president of U of R during the day and I taught yoga evenings and weekends. As a single parent, the supplemental income helped me pay off my home."

Bonnie didn't travel much for trainings. Instead, she faithfully used Friedel Khattab's ten-week class plans and the personal experience she had from healing her own back problem as her compass. Bonnie also insists the best training she had was what she learned from her students. "They shared their improvements with me and I could see their progress. It was often life-changing."

When Iyengar-style yoga came to Regina in the 1980s, Bonnie sensed a change. "It seemed the yoga community became divided," she says. She preferred to stay with her classical method of teaching with no props, and with emphasis on the body supporting itself in each pose. Her teaching also drew from Feldenkrais body movements, which were popular throughout the 1980s, and her understanding of anatomy, which she occasionally taught at the university.

Perhaps Bonnie's most significant contribution, other than being Regina's second yoga teacher after Lloyd Kreitzer, was to tirelessly petition the U of R's physical education faculty (later named the department of kinesiology) to offer yoga as a credit course. She was successful in this endeavour in 2004, providing a curriculum and testing for the department—it remains there to this day.

Bonnie was a founding member of Saskatchewan Yoga Association in 1977, which established a strong foundation for yoga in the province. Now retired and living in Regina, Bonnie says, "Over a period of thirty-five years of teaching, there were endless rewards. I loved the concentration it gave me. My teaching became my meditation. I seldom thought of outside problems when I was teaching. I think everyone needs a passion, no matter how big or small, and this was mine. It kept me in good physical condition and it fixed my back pain. I was always the student and yoga kept me thirsty for more."

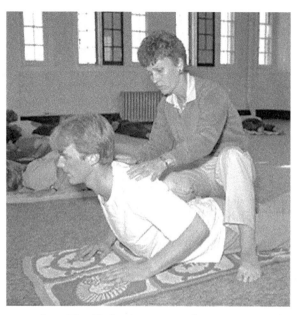

Bonnie Skinner teaching Blair Taylor, University of Regina, 1987. Photo: Dan Hall

Elisabeth Smith

Born Manchester, England 1951 –

Elisabeth immigrated to Canada in 1958 and was introduced to yoga in 1967 at age sixteen in Toronto. She read one of the few yoga books available at the time, *Yoga, Youth and Reincarnation,* by Jess Stearn. Says Elisabeth: "I loved this book. My sister used to say I was a reincarnated yogi, as I used to do yoga poses before I knew what they were. More importantly, I was seeking a spiritual experience and this was confirmation to me that a magical, mystical aspect to life truly did exist beyond just the everyday humdrum. In the late 1960s in Toronto, there was a group of us 'hippies' searching for peace of mind and an alternative lifestyle. I practiced it all, chanting, meditation, whatever was available. For me, yoga satisfied my desire for the mystical more than anything else."

From self-taught, Elisabeth enrolled in classes at the YWCA in Toronto in 1969. She was part of the Kundalini Yoga community of Yogi Bhajan's 3HO Foundation, sought out workshops in the Sivananda method, and started to teach small groups of friends and acquaintances at no charge. She devoured every book she could get her hands on to supplement her training, including those by Richard Hittleman, Kareen Zebroff, and Paramahansa Yogananda.

She arrived in Regina in 1973 and set up classes at the YWCA, community centres, the Regina Public Library, the Legislative Buildings, and the University of Regina, where she taught for nineteen years. She drove to outlying rural towns to introduce yoga to farming communities, inviting them back to Regina for workshops. She was a founding member of the Saskatchewan Yoga Association in 1977, and she was the first to produce videos and cassette tapes to fill the need for yoga instruction at the time.

Elisabeth opened the first yoga business in Regina in 1988, calling it Body/Mind Fitness 1988, and opened various studio spaces. She was the first to give small, intimate yoga retreats, choosing the beautiful setting of the Qu'Appelle Valley, Saskatchewan. Here, she taught yoga, meditation, and visualisation, and cooked the nourishing food herself. Says Elisabeth: "I find preparing meals for people a karmic act of service—food is love and brings community together.

"Seeing people blossom from these teachings is what I most loved. I witnessed how it improved every aspect of their lives. After more than forty years I am now retired, but I keep a daily practice. Like most people, I have had many ups and downs, personal traumas, and difficulties. But throughout it all has been my spiritual path of yoga. It has never failed to keep me calm, relaxed, and centred," says Elisabeth. She lives on Vancouver Island in a home facing the ocean. Here, she gazes out contently from her mat, anchored solidly in the mystic.

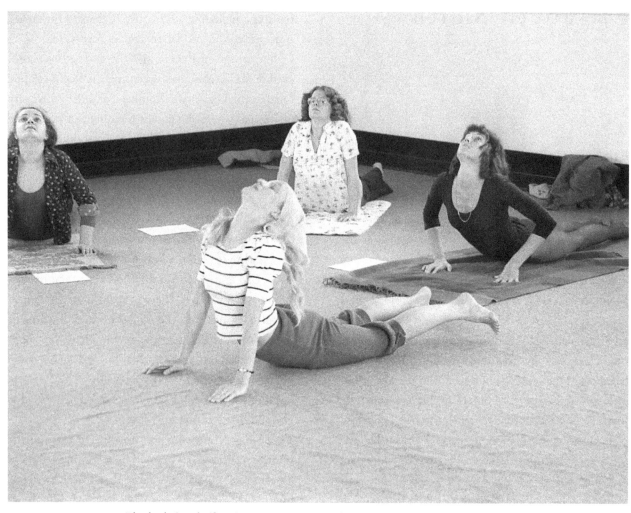

Elisabeth Smith (front), 1975, University of Regina. Photo: Len Middelkamp

Lillian Strauss

Born Biellawa,Poland, 1946 –

At over fifty years, Lillian is Yukon's longest-serving yoga teacher. She picked up yoga just the way you would expect from a true Canadian pioneer—self-taught and living in a shack in the bush! You could say she has true grit.

Lillian immigrated to Toronto from Poland with her parents after World War II. She suffered from scoliosis, crooked feet, and rickets as a child. Despite this, she excelled athletically, earning a dance scholarship with the Toronto Dance Theatre.

But her heart lay in exploring the north. She earned a teaching degree and taught English as a second language to Ojibway children at Whitedog, Ontario, for four years. In 1970, she moved to Whitehorse, Yukon Territory. In addition to loving nature, one of her dreams was to learn to ride horses. A self-professed hippie of her era, she lived in a shack on what is now the Yukon Game Preserve.

"The Yukon cast its spell on me the first summer I arrived. The land, the sky, the rivers, the mountains, the rawness, and the wildness—it's what has kept me here. The Yukon gave me the opportunity to confront my fears—the lessons I needed to learn and am still learning in this life. She gave me an opportunity to grow deep roots. And, yes, I did learn how to ride horses."

Soon after her arrival there, she found BKS Iyengar's book Light on Yoga. Says Lillian: "It became my yoga bible and an exploration for my life-long practice. I attribute healing and miraculous changes in my body to many years of practice from this book. My practice supported me physically, emotionally, and spiritually, and allowed me to give birth to my first two children naturally at home."

Lillian eventually felt confident enough in her practice to teach and started teaching at the YWCA in 1973. She followed with classes in schools, daycares, at the local pool, and at the early studio location above the Alpine Bakery.

When Jeannie Stevens arrived in the Yukon in 1980, they joined together to bring in outside senior teachers to conduct workshops. They always filled to capacity. These teachers were often American friends whose visits helped give the Yukon visibility and included Felicity Green, Judith Lasater, and Rodney Yee. "They really put the Yukon on the map!" says Lillian. They inspired Lillian and Jeannie and other teachers to advance their own practices and move yoga forward in the community, which they did successfully. Eventually, Jeannie moved to Victoria, becoming an author and teacher on yoga for people with ALS and MS. Lillian remained in the Yukon, writing a regular column in *What's Up* magazine, called "Yoga Off the Mat." She continues to teach and devote herself to the growth of yoga in her community.

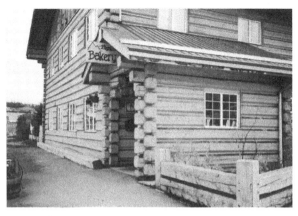

Whitehorse Yoga Studio above Alpine Bakery.
Photo: Jeannie Stevens

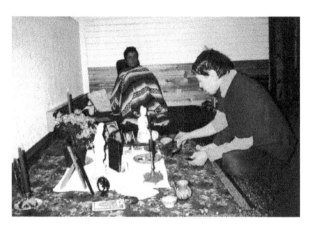

Lillian Strauss sets up altar, Yukon, 1980

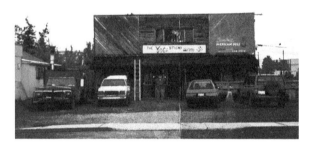

Yukon graduates to Yoga Studio. Photo:
Jeannie Stevens

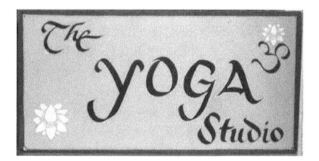

Doris Tobias

Born St. John, New Brunswick, 1929 –

Doris is New Brunswick's quintessential yoga pioneer. Her first exposure to yoga was through a book by Eve Diskin and Eugene Rowls that she picked up on a sale table in the 1960s. She had blood pressure problems and the book assured good health. She read it cover to cover and became a self-taught practitioner. To her, it felt like a hand-and-glove fit. At the same time, she opened a natural foods and vitamin store in Saint John, New Brunswick. In a not-uncommon story with budding yoga teachers, she found herself thrust into teaching when the regular teacher didn't show up for her yoga class at the local YWCA. She was keen to bolster her confidence as a teacher so took training in Val Morin, Quebec, with Swami Vishnudevananda.

Doris taught at various locations in Saint John, such as the Institute for the Blind, St. Paul's Anglican Church in Rothesay, and the Recreation Centre at Gondola Point. Typical of the times, she did not charge for her classes. Money to buy props was often raised through her summer Yoga Yard Sale, which continues today. She started charging five dollars per class when she opened her own studio, The Yoga Room, at Ricky's Mall in Saint John.

Doris defied New Brunswick's reputation as being somewhat sleepy and even behind the times by upgrading her trainings at the Satchidananda Institute in Yogaville, Florida, and Kripalu Center in Lennox, Massachusetts, and returning to share the latest trends.

She met BKS Iyengar in Portland, Maine, on his first trip to America, which kindled an interest and led her to study with Marlene Mawhinney at the Yoga Centre Toronto. Although she represented her home province of New Brunswick at the US Iyengar conference in 1991, Doris states: "I loved Iyengar, but not his harsh methods." However, she did go to the Iyengar Yoga Institute in Pune, India, with Bruce and Maureen Carruthers in 1993 to study.

Doris had heart surgery in May 2018, at the age of eighty-nine. Her recovery was so swift, the doctors said, "We have never met anyone like you. What's your secret?" This petite, demure woman immediately answered, "It's yoga!" Doris swiftly returned to teaching and is supported by a group of loyal, long-term students. Not surprisingly, she is directing her energy toward assisting those with heart issues.

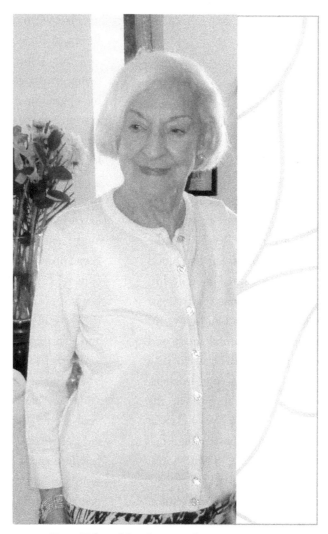

Doris Tobias, New Brunswick pioneer, age 89

Jessica Tucker

Born Chennai (then Madras), India, 1914; died Victoria, British Columbia, 2012

From a British boarding school in Tamil Nadu, India, to nursing in a hospital in London, England, to sailing in Vancouver, Canada, Jessica was a progressive woman for her time.

She was one of the first three teachers in Vancouver in the mid-1960s and the first to introduce yoga to the YWCA in Victoria, which grew to twenty-five classes and spread yoga to Vancouver Island.

Her psychiatrist husband was an avid sailor, but Jessica's fear of water held her back from enjoying it with him. She set out to do something about it by enrolling in yoga classes with Bina Nelson at the YWCA in Vancouver. Not only did she learn yogic breathing to deal with her anxiety, she came away with an intense passion to learn more. She became good friends with Bina, learning everything she could and reading voraciously. At Bina's encouragement, she jumped in and started to teach.

Her husband was transferred to Victoria in 1967, and once there Jessica lost no time in approaching the YWCA to convince them to set up yoga classes. The practice of yoga was suspect at the time, and the YWCA, as a Christian organization, was apprehensive about the public perception of yoga as a cult. Despite the fact that Jessica was a strict Roman Catholic who used yoga to deepen her own faith, they nevertheless asked her to call it a "psychomotor exercise" class. One year later, after a favourable response, they switched to naming it what it was—yoga. Thanks to forward-thinking people and Jessica's tenacity, the classes flourished. She taught women-only classes first, then also to men and children. She started training teachers to meet the demand, all of them volunteering their time.

She felt it was important for students to know there was a philosophy to yoga so she would bring in charts to the classroom outlining Patanjali's Eight Limbs of Yoga.

Jessica would not accept pay for teaching. Says her daughter Penny: "She held a strong belief in the 1950s version of the 'ideal family.' She believed that married women should look after their homes, their gardens, and their dogs. Volunteer work was OK, but having a paid job was not. She gave talks about this at the YWCA and was not very impressed that my sister and I both had careers!"

Jessica taught at the Y in Victoria until 1975, at which time she had a hip replacement and never went back. Says Penny: "I think she was afraid that doing yoga would damage her new hip." Jessica went on to become a mature student at University of Victoria when she was well into her sixties, studying art history and philosophy. She later became wheelchair-bound from a Parkinson's-like disorder.

When she was in her early nineties, she had a stroke. "It was evident her years of practicing yoga helped her cope with this and gave her the calm she had always sought," says Penny.

Jessica is noted as a pioneer who helped launch yoga in British Columbia and who helped break down misconceptions around it. She died in 2012 at age ninety-eight in Victoria.

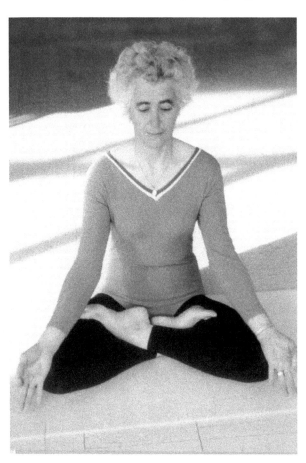

Jessica Tucker, Vancouver, 1967

Jutta Wiedemann

Born Bad Salzuflen, Germany, 1930 –

Jutta was the third teacher in Vancouver, starting in 1967. Jutta and colleague Pegge Gabbott are recognized as the founding members of the Hatha Yoga Teachers Association, British Columbia's first yoga teacher's organization. It was incorporated under the Societies Act in 1971.

Jutta first attended classes with Jessica Tucker in West Vancouver in search of relief from her back problems. Getting good results, she went directly to Jessica's teacher, Bina Nelson, and asked for training. Eager to teach, she called on the school boards in Vancouver and Surrey, offering to set up classes. At the time there was still a lot of skepticism about yoga. Says Jutta: "They would usually ask for a few days to think about it, which meant they couldn't get agreement on whether to take the leap, but luckily, they called back and said yes. Once I got my foot in the door, there was no looking back. People really wanted to know what yoga was about. From there, I added community centres and churches, and I had all the classes I wanted."

Jutta and Pegge were forward thinkers, advocating vegetarianism along with yoga before it was a trend. The advent of yoga was not without its critics, however. Some local religious extremists were against it. When Jutta and her friend Kareen Zebroff and others were accused of "witchcraft" by these preachers, they were officially summoned to Vancouver City Hall. They defended themselves by providing education on what yoga was. Kareen also used her substantial writing skills and published a rebuttal in *Common Ground* magazine: "Yoga is not a religion, but rather an art, science, and philosophy that helps us cope with our stressed out modern existence so that we might maximize our potential as human beings."

Jutta went to study at the Iyengar Institute in India in 1979, claiming her trip to India was one of the peak experiences in her life.

In the 1980s, while suffering a migraine while on a holiday in Germany, it was discovered that Jutta had a brain tumour. She had a successful surgery and recovery, which she credits to her knowledge and lifelong practice of yoga asana, meditation, and visualization.

The HYTA is no longer active, but many of its members still meet every summer at Yellow Point Lodge on Vancouver Island for practice and fellowship, as they have for over forty years. At ninety years old, Jutta often helps organize these meetings.

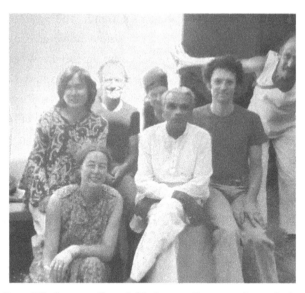

Jutta Wiedemann (front left), Iyengar Institute, Pune, India

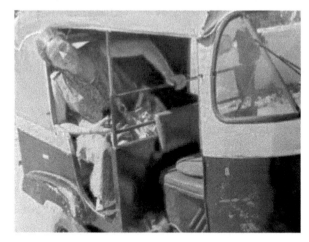

Jutta Wiedemann, India, 1979

Part 3
Trailblazers

Within this section are those who were inspired by the Searchers of the 1960s and '70s, and often dovetailed with them, creatively adding to the rich tapestry of yoga in Canada. During the 1980s, provincial associations, cable TV stations, libraries, and visiting Americans were still the primary source for learning about yoga. Communities continued to form. A few bold conferences were organized here and there across the country. A handful of commercial (for-profit) yoga studios began to open. Then, all of a sudden, in the late 1990s, the growth of yoga took on the speed of a freight train, with some statistics touting it as the fastest-growing industry in North America. A businessman bought the non-profit *Yoga Journal* magazine in 1998, and soon after went digital. Various hybrids of yoga asana styles started to emerge. Lululemon Athletica's Chip and Shannon Wilson propelled the yoga culture forward not only by making fun yoga wear but also by including yoga teachers across Canada as "ambassadors" to their meaningful philanthropic network. Meditation found its stride with the Science of Meditation on the cover of *Time* magazine in 2001. Yoga and meditation became a prescription for everything from back problems to depression. Without enough teachers to meet the demand, Canada's yoga trailblazers found themselves at the forefront of this phenomenon. They saw unique opportunities to facilitate new pathways of understanding. They were indeed the bridge-builders of yoga and meditation, introducing it into medical, corporate, and educational settings.

Francine Cauchy

Born Seine-St-Denis, France, 1942 –

When Francine began experiencing depression after the loss of her father in 1965, a friend suggested she try yoga. She followed that advice and was soon hooked, studying as much as she could outside of her daytime work as a school teacher.

She started yoga classes with Anne de Couessin in Paris, who learned from André Van Lysebeth, author of *Yoga Self-Taught*. She also studied with Noëlle Perez, who, in 1959, became one of the first Western students to study with BKS Iyengar. It was Noëlle who encouraged Francine to become a teacher.

Francine pursued her passion when she immigrated to Montreal in 1975 to attend the Lotus Center for the Development of Being, founded by Claude Passaro (Swami Shraddananda). She became a teacher in the Sivananda tradition and was initiated with the name Madhura in 1977. She stayed at the LCDB as co-director, teacher, and trainer for twelve years.

Francine returned to France in 1988 and resumed being a schoolteacher and then school principal. Influenced by the trend she saw in other European countries, she began to successfully integrate yoga into the French school system. She simultaneously pursued a diploma in Ayurveda at the European Institute of Vedic Studies and an advanced course with Dr. David Frawley of the European Institute. This period of study, meditation, and asceticism on the links between yoga, ayurveda (Eastern medicine) and jyotish (astrology) was to prove instrumental in helping Francine define her life path.

Francine returned to Quebec in 2005. She settled in Mont-Saint-Hilaire on the Richelieu River, where she established the Vidya Institute. Here, she launched classes in *yoga nidra* (yogic sleep), *prana vidya* (science of breath), ayurveda, and yoga for seniors and children. Her work with yoga and children especially took bloom.

Francine says: "I have observed the benefits of yoga on children. Yoga has improved their posture. They are more attentive in class, both quieter and better centred. Their relationships are happier. Kids today spend too much time on their screens and tablets. Studies confirm that this activity has adverse effects on their minds. Children are criticized for lack of attention and concentration and for physically being either too apathetic or hyperactive. Yoga helps them rebalance these effects, roots them, allows them to inhabit their bodies differently, and develop attention and concentration. They reconnect with who they are in deep within."

Her trainings were timely and well received in Quebec. Her book, *Guide to Help the Child Grow, Succeed and Flourish,* offers simple yoga routines for children and is a useful manual for parents. She works under the Federation of Francophone Yoga to train yoga teachers for educational organizations.

A researcher, trainer, teacher, and author of books and articles, Francine laid the groundwork for yoga in the schools in Quebec. She is advisor for the World Council of Yoga and became an honorary member of the FFY in 2015 after fifty years of service to others through yoga. She inspired her three children on the path of yoga and her son Raphael teaches with her at the Vidya Institute.

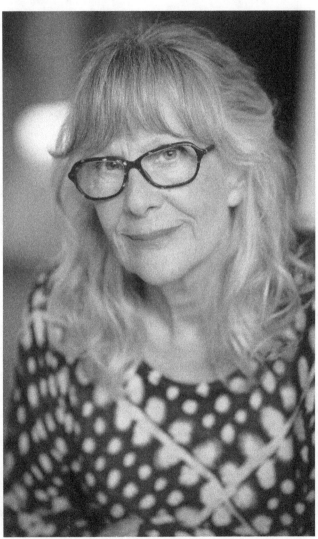

Francine Cauchy, yoga pioneer and educator, Quebec

Janice Clarfield

Born Toronto, Ontario, 1952 –

Janice was the first teacher to create a prenatal yoga teacher training program in western Canada. It went on to gain international recognition and launch hundreds of prenatal teachers. Her teachings are the result of her own personal struggles—she dealt with depression all her life. She grew up in Toronto in a family with a strict upbringing and painful roots in the Holocaust. Janice knew she had to leave, and in August 1971, she ran away to Vancouver, where she knew no one. It was a leap of faith into the unknown that was to characterize Janice's entire life. She moved into an apartment in Kitsilano and immersed herself in the alternative culture of the time.

She started to wear flowing clothes, she played Joni Mitchell , and she sought out yoga. She attended her first yoga class at Vancouver's original studio with Bina Nelson and later with Maureen Tribe (later Carruthers) at the Unitarian church on Oak Street. Then came an opportunity to study with Joel Kramer at Cold Mountain Institute (later known as Hollyhock Retreat) on Cortes Island. It was here that she experienced a certainty that this was her life's path.

Says Janice: "Yoga and meditation have saved my life. Even in utero I was close to the existential dilemma. In suffering depression, I questioned the mystery of what it is to be a human being. Yoga and meditation provided a crucible of refuge. It provided a safe place for me to deepen that inquiry. I believe consciousness starts in the womb and the gestation process is sacred."

After taking Sandra Sammartino's teacher training in the early 1980s, Janice opened Vancouver's fifth studio, Urban Yoga. As so often happens in life, it is our painful past that defines our future, and this was true for Janice. Lamenting over never having a child and still exploring her own in-utero experience, she felt an affinity with expectant mothers. She vividly recalls an evening where she had a pregnant student in her class and was wondering how to serve her better for the upcoming childbirth. What was needed to assist her in this important experience? How could she be authentic? Says Janice, "I am not a mother, yet somehow I felt I had a lot to offer them. My fascination with pregnancy, the birth process, and new life kept drawing me. Not having a child is a sorrow for me, so how could I be there for the miracle when it touched my own loss? I knew in my bones and heart that I had something to offer."

Flooded with inspiration and research, Janice filled her prenatal classes and wrote and launched *Conscious and Sacred Birthing*. Her work was timely and people were keen to hear this spiritual dimension being discussed in childbirth preparation. Says Janice of her work: "My work is about creating optimum conditions for the next generation to be birthed as wisely, compassionately, and consciously as possible. Modern neural brain science says formation of the brain is impacted and this affects humanity. Pregnant women who are in environments that are peaceful, loving, and safe, have babies whose brains are inclined toward wholesome human qualities. I call this spiritual component 'sacred birthing.' Is there anything more important than how we bring in the next generation? My approach was and is yogic and holistic. Be present, be grounded. Be centred and balanced."

Janice was soon doing ten trainings a year internationally. She was interviewed by radio and TV stations on *Conscious Birthing* and appeared in publications such as *Yoga Journal* in Japan. Most prenatal trainings in Canada today can be traced to her work.

Janice turned her personal loss into her life work and her sorrow into a joy by participating wholeheartedly and joyfully in the birth of a generation. She has retired from trainings, but continues to write and accept speaking invitations.

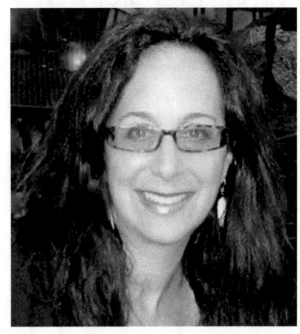

Janice Clarfield

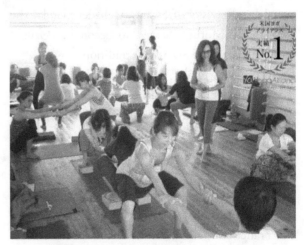

Janice Clarfield training teachers, Japan

Karen Fletcher

Born Winnipeg, Manitoba, 1954 –

When Karen was in high school in Winnipeg in 1970, she overheard two girls talking about yoga. Says Karen: "I felt a tingling feeling going up and down my spine. I knew there was something in it for me." It was a premonition of her remarkable journey ahead being the first to bring yoga and meditation to nursing in Manitoba.

She started classes at the YMCA and later held yoga philosophy classes with scholar Ranen Sinha. Encouraged by Ranen to teach, and further influenced by the visits of Swami Mahadevananda, she went to Val Morin, Quebec, to become a certified yoga teacher in the Sivananda tradition.

Years later, when her girlfriend Louise was dying of breast cancer, Karen was a constant by her bedside. She found it natural to give her comfort and she found clarity of purpose, remarking to her good friend Sheri Berkowitz, "This is what I want to do with my life."

Louise's death plunged Karen into a deep inquiry about life and death. As part of her quest, she went to San Francisco to live at the Sivananda ashram while earning a master's degree in east/west psychology at the Institute of Integral Studies. Her friend Sheri was also in San Francisco at that time studying at the Iyengar Institute. Intrigued by this new method, they practiced it together and introduced it to the Winnipeg yoga community upon their return home.

When her sister came to visit and talked about her experiences in palliative care nursing, Karen again felt that deep resonance, knowing this was the next step in her calling. Upon returning from studies at the Iyengar Institute in Pune, India, in 1985, she signed up for nursing school at the University of Manitoba and began her groundbreaking work of introducing yoga to the medical community.

Becoming director of nursing at Cancer Care Manitoba, Karen began teaching palliative care to nursing students at the University of Manitoba. Radical for its time, she started each class with a meditation and grounding. She taught them how to practice quietness and presence before they walked in to see a patient. Says Karen: "You have to move into a place where you are not panicking, not trying to fix anything, but rather experiencing things as they come and go, building that capacity to be with someone who is suffering or dying. Yes, you have to be good at managing pain, that is a given, but more important is the loving, still presence. This comes only by being present to our own suffering first."

Karen impressed upon her trainees that they could only have the stamina to be a quiet presence if they had a personal practice. Yoga and meditation in Winnipeg were still in their infancy and little understood. Karen credits a supportive and forward-thinking organization at the University of Manitoba for encouraging her work in those early years.

Karen was a senior teacher at the Yoga Studio Winnipeg when it opened. She was also the first, along with teacher Val Paape, to launch classes for cancer patients, and she led them faithfully for over ten years.

Karen's foresight in introducing yoga skills like savasana (relaxation) and guided meditation into nursing brought the spiritual dimension of the death process into the open. She spent her last few years in palliative care teaching a death assistance care plan during her rounds with doctors and social workers.

Karen's legacy also includes a published professional paper called *Midwifing Distress at End of Life*. These were tips she drew from her personal experience in coping with her husband's early death and, later, her mother's death, which she describes as "Nothing short of a miracle process —from extreme resistance to Grace."

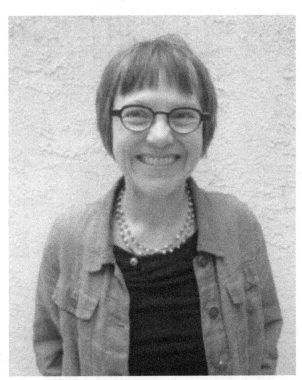

Karen Fletcher, Winnipeg, Manitoba teaches yoga for palliative care

Ted Grand

Born Toronto, Ontario, 1968 –

Ted is co-founder of the first cross-Canada chain of yoga studios, Modo Yoga (formerly Moksha Yoga). His yoga chain changed the landscape of yoga in Canada by including environmental and community stewardship as requirements for ownership. His legacy is substantial and hard won.

It began with personal transformation. As a youth, he was sensitive to suffering in the world and strove to change what he saw as injustices around him. Becoming an activist in several global and local organizations, he gave it his all. He often felt he was racing against time. The more he saw, the angrier and more helpless he felt, so the more he pushed. There were two arrests. There were relationship breakdowns, and always a deep, lingering frustration. And then he found yoga.

Says Ted of choosing yoga: "It was a concerted effort at cultivating more peace in my life. The intensity of the work I had been doing for the environment—animal rights, and anti-poverty and human rights work— had left me feeling overwhelmed and alone. For every step forward it felt like there were several steps back, and after a while it seemed like I was becoming more and more removed from my heart, and a simmering anger began to boil. It was meditation and yoga that brought me a deeper understanding that I can transform that anger and harness it to bring more peace into my life and into the world."

He took his first yoga class in Whistler in 1994, and thereafter jumped in with characteristic passion, seeing yoga as a doorway to the higher consciousness he sought for the world.

While in Toronto for two years to be with his ill mother, he practiced regularly at the Downward Dog Yoga Studio. Then he attended the University of Santa Cruz in California to study organic farming. To put it to the test, he moved to Nelson, British Columbia, where he grew his own food while living on a mountain with no electricity, creating an environment for him to deepen his practice. When his girlfriend handed him a sheet of Bikram yoga poses, he practiced vigorously, eventually going to Los Angeles to get certified with Bikram Choudhury. Teaching Bikram's method exclusively, he opened his first studio, Yaletown Yoga, in Vancouver in 2001.

Ted and fellow activist and yoga teacher Jessica Robertson met and teamed up to open a brand of yoga studios that included a focus on community outreach and the environment. They started with Bikram studios in Toronto, Danforth, Oakville, and London, Ontario. About this time, Bikram was attempting to enforce strict copyright policies on his studios and Ted disagreed. The relationship severed. An evolutionary curve had begun. Ted had already realized that a stringent sequence of twenty-six poses was mechanical, falling short of meeting each person at their level of need. He flew to Pune, India, to study with physician Dr. Karandikar—a longtime protégé of BKS Iyengar—and learned a larger repertoire of carefully sequenced poses to address individual needs.

Jessica and Ted co-founded and trademarked the name Moksha Yoga for their studios in 2004, and stayed with the hot yoga theme established by Bikram. When interest came from the US, they adopted the name *Modo Yoga*, and began opening studios there with copartners. Today, the name has changed from Moksha to Modo and there are over seventy studios worldwide.

Not wanting a traditional business model that included rapid expansion for its own sake, Ted and Jessica were firmly committed to one that focused primarily on building conscious community, engaging environmental stewardship, and generating revenue for non-profit causes through its karma classes. To date, Modo Yoga has raised over five million dollars for organizations such as crisis centres, shelters, and prisons.

With strict criteria for entry, more applicants for studio ownership are refused than accepted. Although most franchisors would shudder at this way of doing business, Ted and Jessica believe the values over profit approach ensure quality control and, more importantly, is in line with their personal values. Today, they have carved out separate duties within their organization that allow each to express their strengths. Both screen all the applicants and oversee their vision of yoga as a compassionate vehicle for nothing less than planetary change.

As so often happens with successful businesses, the Modo concept is being emulated everywhere. To them, it simply strengthens their commitment to lead responsibly. Their goal is to create a chain reaction of conscious living for a better world—for them, it exemplifies the yoga path.

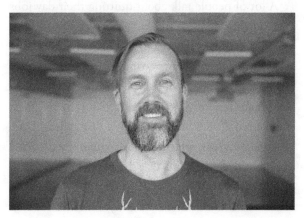

Ted Grand, co-founder, Moda (Moksha) Yoga

Kelly Green

Born Regina, Saskatchewan, 1958 –

A lot of people talk about quitting their day jobs and starting a yoga studio. Kelly actually did it, opening the first yoga studio in Regina in 1993. She also started Regina's first commercial yoga teacher training program. More importantly, as Kelly's understanding of yoga as a sacred process grew, she offered classes and workshops that reflected the spiritual element. Her life work culminated in the one-of-a-kind programs that she offers in Regina.

Kelly began by practicing yoga from Richard Hittleman's book *Yoga: 28 Day Exercise Plan* in 1973. She then started practicing along with Kareen Zebroff on TV. Says Kelly of Kareen: "She was so exotic, so inviting, she made me feel 'I can do this!'"

In her career as a medical social worker (psychosocial support for people with health issues), Kelly believed that yoga could help people reach their potential and was keen to bridge the two worlds of yoga and medical social work. Like so many others early on, she sought out trainings with American teachers. She studied with Felicity Green in Bellingham and iRest creator Richard Miller in California. She became certified as a Relax and Renew trainer with Judith Lasater of San Francisco and graduated from the school of Integrative Yoga Therapy in Marin County, California. She immersed herself in mindfulness meditation trainings with Shirley Johannesen and Thich Nhat Hanh. All the while, she introduced many of these teachings to Regina.

Kelly was social worker by day and a yoga teacher by night until she took a leap of faith in 1993 to devote herself full time to her new yoga studio, named Inward Bound, later changed to Prairie Yoga Studio. She invited senior teachers from all over Canada and the US to come and teach, enticing them with her prairie hospitality.

For Kelly, her various trainings converged to one point—helping students in their transformational processes. Seeing her role as a facilitator for the sacred awakening that often arises with the ardent student, she chose to strengthen those skills by certifying as a life coach. Says Kelly: "Rumi says that love's greatest gift is its ability to make everything it touches sacred. It has been, and continues to be, my intention to offer spiritual practices for everyday lives. I aspire to spark others to sparkle as the most conscious, whole versions of themselves."

Today, Kelly teaches classes called Living Yoga, or what she refers to as "taking the mat into daily life." In these teachings she takes students through various practices of asana, pranayama, the timeless Eight Limbs of Yoga philosophy, and meditation.

She changed her company name one last time to Every Day Sacred. Says Kelly: "I wanted a name that would reflect where I was authentically with guiding my students to explore the sacred in all they do. As a 'recovering perfectionist,' I know firsthand the value of celebrating where we are, right now, no conditions, and it all stems from the practice of yoga and our acknowledging our spiritual perfection."

Kelly offered Wonder Woman's Wisdom and More than a Mom circles as themes for women to meet, share their wisdom, and grow consciously. She now offers classes for mid-years women called Becoming Ageless Sages. These classes incorporate spiritual psychology and soul-centred coaching. Kelly became ordained as an interfaith minister so she could design and facilitate rituals and ceremonies to assist people in celebrating life's milestones, such as weddings, celebrations of life, and baby blessings. She believes that the process of spiritual inquiry and expression is more alive when it involves celebrating life's stages.

Kelly's success meant trusting herself to grow from studio owner and teacher trainer to life minister, coach, and guru. Kelly jokes, "I call myself the 'love guru.' I often sign, 'Rev. Kelly, cheerleader of the heart' after my name or when I sign posts."

Her programs would not have happened without believing in her creativity. She continues to give programs that help others navigate life's changes using yoga and meditation as guideposts. She could not have done this without being grounded in the sacred through her own practice and being willing to boldly follow the direction of her calling.

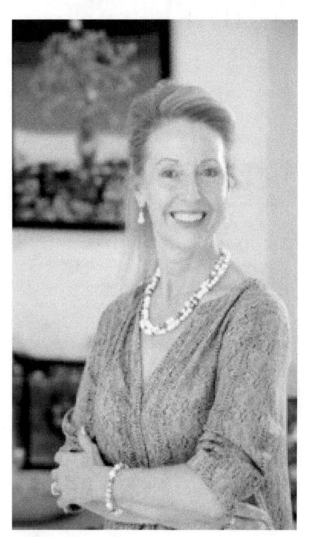

Kelly Green, first yoga studio, Regina, Saskatchewan

Ida Herbert

Born England, 1916 –

The world's oldest yoga teacher in the *Guinness Book of World Records* is none other than a Canadian who hails from Orillia, Ontario.

Ida emigrated from England in 1948 with her husband. To date, no other Canadian has beat her record. Calling herself a late bloomer, Ida was in her early fifties when she found yoga. "I was at the gym, cycling away on the phony bicycle, and I saw a girl against the mirrors," Herbert says. "I asked the assistant, 'What's that lady doing over there?'"

The woman informed her it was yoga and Ida got interested. She picked up Kareen Zebroff's book, *The ABC of Yoga*, laid it face open on her living room floor, and started to practice. She was hooked!

She wasn't daunted by her lack of formal training and began teaching at the local YMCA in Orillia.

With her trademark sense of humour, Ida was a big hit and she attracted a strong following that stuck with her through the years. Her loyal ladies showed their commitment by showing up with T-shirts that said "Ida's Girls," and the name stuck. Undeterred by the onset of age-related macular degeneration, an eye disease that deteriorates vision, Ida remained the loyal teacher to her 'girls,' emphatically stating her well known mantra, "Move, girls, move!" Years later, the YMCA was to bestow her with an honorary certificate.

She was nominated the world's oldest yoga teacher at age ninety-six due to the eagle eye of eleven-year-old Kobe Rose, whose mom, Rosanna Shililo, is also a yoga teacher in Orillia. In 2012, while poring over an old edition of the *Guinness Book of World Records*, he noticed the world's oldest yoga teacher was listed as a ninety-year-old teacher from the UK. He remembered seeing a newspaper article about Ida in his mom's studio and contacted officials at Guinness. The title was transferred to Ida, who remained actively teaching until age ninety-six. The title has brought a lot of publicity Ida's way and she has delighted in it. Often asked if she had any other secrets to longevity besides yoga, Ida remarks: "I have a positive attitude. I don't let any bugs in," clarifying that she meant bad thoughts. "And my fondness for sherry seems to have paid off," she adds with a giggle.

When Ida turned 100 on August 21, 2016, she was given a birthday party by her wellwishers and Ida's Girls, hosted by the YMCA. She now lives in a retirement home in Orillia, where she still practices what she can and you can occasionally hear her mantra echo through the halls—*"Move girls, move!"* followed by her famous laugh.

Yoga instructor, 95, goes for Guinness

Ida Herbert in the running for world's oldest yoga teacher title

LISA MIRIAM CHERRY
SPECIAL TO THE STAR

"We're going to do the Hula," 95-year-old Ida Herbert shouts out to the packed yoga class at Breathe Yoga Studio in Toronto's Junction area. "Let it go, girls!"

Dressed in black tights and a navy leotard, Herbert swirls an imaginary hoop around her tiny 4'10" frame. The 50 female clients, aged from 30 to 70, follow her lead.

It's warm-up time, Ida Herbert-style. Next Herbert wraps her legs in rock-the-baby pose, crossing them over her chest to hug them in. She implores everyone else to do the same and "get the fluid around the cartilage moving."

"Don't let it sit there — take a breath and enjoy yoga," she says encouragingly as she raises her arms and legs into the v-seated boat pose for five-minutes. It's a move that's arduous even when you're many years younger.

Herbert has been a yoga practitioner for 45 years and a teacher for the past 20. The former secretary, who was born in England during World War I and came to Canada with her late husband Michael after World War II, regularly teaches yoga to a dedicated group known as Ida's Girls at her Bayshore Village housing complex, near Orillia.

She was invited to teach the special workshop and share her years of wisdom at Breathe studio.

Ida's Girls and the folks at Breathe are not Herbert's only followers. Guinness World Records is currently assessing her claim to be the oldest living yoga instructor, said Jamie Panas, public relations manager at Guinness World Records NA, Inc. "Since we announced Ber-

nice Bates (91) as the oldest yoga instructor last November, we've been flooded with applications for this title," Panas said. The successful candidate will be announced at the end of the summer and recorded in the *Guinness World Records 2013* book, which launches Sept. 13.

Herbert discovered yoga in the 1960s, long before Angela Farmer invented the yoga mat or *Kareen's Yoga* hit the television airwaves in the '70s.

As a 50-year-old school secretary in Toronto, Herbert, who "quite disliked exercising," had never heard

about yoga until she spotted a woman teaching asanas in a hotel gym one day. "What on earth is that?" she recalls thinking. "It looked so nice. I had to learn more."

After asking around, Herbert discovered she'd been watching yoga and enlisted a friend, who was taking classes, to teach her at home. She learned a couple of new asanas each week and read books to learn more. Eventually she became a dedicated practitioner — rising at 5:30 every morning for yoga, something she continues to this day.

Little did she know, she was a yogi-

ni pioneer breaking into the historically-patriarchal yogic ranks populated by legendary teachers like Vanda Scaravelli and Indra Devi, masters who lived healthfully past 90 years of age.

"That's what yoga can do for you," Herbert reflects in an almost inaudible whisper. "Your limbs are working but your inside is very peaceful and quiet. It quietened my mind, my body, my senses, my emotions. I realized this one day when I was touching my toes."

Especially peaceful for Herbert is holding asanas for long periods. "I

love all the poses, but have never done headstands. And never will," she says, adding that she prefers to protect her neck.

After retiring in 1986, Ida and Michael started snow-birding in Florida. When the local exercise teacher moved away, Ida began teaching yoga for free. "I fell into it quite naturally. I don't even consider it teaching. I just like to encourage people to do things that are good for themselves."

When the couple moved from Toronto to Orillia, Herbert taught at the local Y, which gave her special certification.

Now, no longer able to drive because she has macular degeneration, the community centre at her housing complex is her primary studio.

"I don't advertise them as yoga classes, however. Just as 'exercise classes' so as not to scare off the men," she jokes. Alas, the men have never shown up. And with the plow and boat poses, the "girls" caught on that it's yoga.

Fifteen years ago, on her 80th birthday, a dozen or so of Ida's students — all women from 60 to 80 years old — arrived at class in shirts emblazoned with "Ida's Girls." The name stuck.

So, is it Herbert's daily yoga practice that's kept her looking seventy-something, with a sharp wit and mind?

"You could attribute some of my longevity to that," she answers. "But I also eat no junk food, love gardening and drink sherry after lunch. Oh, and I love to flirt."

A keen cyclist, Herbert had to stop biking around town two months ago after a bad fall, but she has no plans to give up teaching yoga.

"I plan to go on until my body stops me! Or until my girls do!"

Lisa Miriam Cherry is the editor of Stories from the Yogic Heart, www.yogicheart.com

RICHARD LAUTENS PHOTOS/TORONTO STAR

In Toronto to teach a special yoga class at Breathe studio, Ida Herbert, 95, counsels her "girls" to let it go. "I just like to encourage people to do things that are good for themselves," she says.

Ida Herbert, world's oldest yoga teacher, The Toronto Star 2012

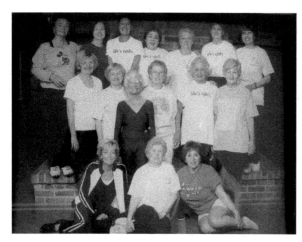

Ida with Ida's Girls, Orillia, Ontario

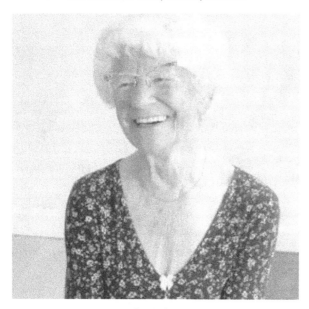

Ida Herbert

Martin Jerry

Born Toronto, Ontario, 1934 –

Marion Jerry

Born Wheatley, Ontario, 1937 –

Martin and Marion met as staff at a summer camp for children with disabilities at Lake Erie, Ontario, in their youth. Their rapport was instant and they sat for long hours talking about the deep spiritual mysteries of the world. Different in temperament, Marion was heart-focused and Martin more cerebral. Yet they were fused by their complementary differences. They were yin and yang.

These two remarkable individuals went on to share a sixty-five-plus-year marriage and leave a lasting legacy to the yoga world through their writings and humanitarian work.

They achieved numerous degrees, Martin as a physician with a PhD in immunology and Marion as a psychologist and nurse. Their career paths always merged for discussion in their mutual interest—spirituality. Their larger metaphysical questions about life still hovered.

After a professorship at McGill University, Martin accepted a position as director of the Southern Alberta Cancer Clinic in Calgary, later called the Tom Baker Cancer Centre. With Calgary as their home, his skills as an oncologist, immune expert, and administrative specialist assisted clinics in Alberta, and, later in life, other clinics through the World Health Organization. Through it all, he remained interested in the effects of spirituality on wellness. Marion started as a psychologist and later became director of psychosocial oncology at Calgary Cancer Centre, where she established a program that provided emotional and social support for patients during treatment—the first of its kind in Canada. It received initial resistance from traditionalists, but paved the way in Calgary for psycho-spiritual care today.

All of these accomplishments served as a platform for their larger work ahead. They explored the Rosicrucians; they attended Transcendental Meditation ® meetings; they delved into neuro-linguistic programming; they visited the Self-Realization Fellowship in Encinitas, California.

And then it all changed. After attending a lecture given by Swami Veda of the Himalayan yoga tradition, they met his master, Swami Rama from the Himalayan Institute in Honesdale, Pennsylvania. They describe this as a fortuitous event that found them committing on the spot to Swami Rama and initiation into the Himalayan tradition.

Says Martin: "There was no hesitation whatsoever as it seemed to us we had arrived at our spiritual destination. Once you have met a master, your life is changed forever. Forces were at work. A door opened and we walked through it, and again, looking back, we could see the whole pattern."

In 1983, they opened up their home to a study group, which became known as the Foothills Yoga

Society. Martin started to do research on meditation with volunteers from the group to show the effect of meditation on immunology. His reports showed how meditation "turns genes on." At that time in his professional field, no one was really interested. Years later, this area would gain interest as psychoneuroimmunology.

Marion and Martin spent summers studying and teaching at the institute's meditation centre in Minneapolis. They also worked at Rishikesh Hospital in India, which was founded under the Himalayan Institute Hospital Trust. Through the Division of International Development at the University of Calgary, Martin was able to acquire a substantial five-year grant from the Canadian International Development Agency as well as funding from Rotary International. The outreach program established brought health care to surrounding villages built on expressed needs for literacy and income generation. The U of C, Tom Baker Cancer Centre, and World Health Organization supported additional programs for pediatrics, oncology, nursing, and dentistry.

Says Marion: "People from villages had to walk forever for help with cancer. Today that has all changed, thanks to people from Calgary."

Martin and Marion published three successive books that synthesized their knowledge as a scientist and psychologist on the spiritual path. "In meditative communion with the centre, the material simply flowed as fast as it could be written down. In New Age jargon, this might be called channeling the 'centre of consciousness.' In the yogic paradigm, it is the intuitive revelation that characterizes communion with the centre," says Martin. "We have great respect for material given in this way—that it be presented as purely as possible. We function simply as messengers, not as teachers who *know*. The words literally flowed onto the page." The first was *Sutras of the Inner Teacher*, which began as a curriculum for the teacher training program at the Himalayan Meditation Center in Minneapolis, and was later adopted into curriculum by the Yoga Studio College of Canada, in Calgary. This was followed by *The Chariots of Sadhana* and *Journey to the Centre*, forming a trilogy that provides a comprehensive spiritual road map for any serious yoga practitioner. Throughout, the centre of consciousness is described as "the essential direct experience."

Says Martin: "Yoga is a science of spirituality. Swami Rama taught it as a science. People get caught up in the ritual, dogma, and religion and miss the basis of it all. You must be able to work from direct experience. It is an evidence-based spirituality."

The Jerrys are now retired and live private lives in Canmore, Alberta. They have two sons—Paul is a psychologist and Mark is a Lutheran pastor and economist. Their last workshop at the Yoga Studio of Calgary in 2001 was described by one participant as "the workshop of the century" because of its cutting-edge content.

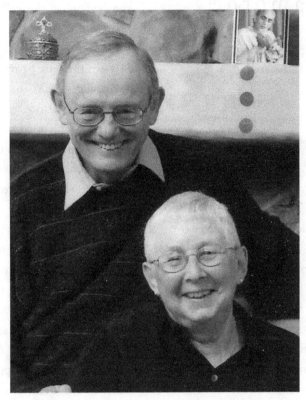

Martin and Marion Jerry, Canmore, Alberta,
personify the joy of living and serving

Christine Lamothe

Born Ottawa, Ontario, 1977 –

Christine opened the first yoga studio in the town of Iqaluit in the territory of Nunavut in 2014. An area of two million square kilometres and accessible only by air or Ski-Doo, it has a population of about 7,000 people. No yoga had ever existed in Nunavut before. None.

Today, Iqaluit is home to Samaivik, an Inuktitut term for "place of peace and tranquility," featuring a team of seven trained teachers and a variety of yoga therapy classes. This is all thanks to a young, spirited woman named Christine Lamothe.

Christine didn't always have a feeling of tranquility. "I was a tough chick," she says. "I was a break-dancer and I learned on the streets in Ottawa. I had bouts of depression and suicidal thoughts when I was young. In 1998, I met a yoga teacher who encouraged me to try Bikram yoga as athletic and challenging." Taking that advice, she started classes with Ed Hum in Ottawa and enthusiastically embraced yoga. She then got interested in the deeper, esoteric aspects of yoga and took kundalini yoga training. Before long, she was rising at four-thirty every morning for a *sadhana* (spiritual) practice. During this time,

she had what she calls "a profound, spontaneous *kundalini* experience." Her bouts of depression and suicidal thoughts disappeared and confirmed for her this was the only path she needed.

In March 2006, she was invited to go to Nunavut as part of a breakdance crew to teach high school kids and she leapt at the opportunity. Maybe, just maybe, there would be an opening to talk about yoga? The event was successful, and there was an invitation for more projects to engage youth and reduce drug abuse and suicide. Christine saw a chance to do something really worthwhile—to help youth who were experiencing what she had come through, and to introduce yoga. She jumped in. Thinking of ways to launch, Christine purchased an old orange building to turn into a yoga studio. To start her business, she took money from the sale of her condo in Ottawa and a small business loan from Baffin Business Development. Says Christine: "I didn't want to do the non-profit approach. For me, doing it as a business was the most expedient and effective way to get the job done. I took all the risks. I didn't want to rely on other people. In total I spent $100,000 of my own money. I felt a need to prove to the locals I was not just another white girl showing up to make money in the north. I genuinely wanted to help, and I knew personally the transformative power of yoga."

Christina visited the Home Depot in Montreal and purchased $30,000 in supplies. Since access to Iqaluit is only by plane for most of the year, the shipping costs came to an additional $13,000. The end result? A charming orange building turned yoga studio in Iqaluit with hardwood floors, a prayer bowl, and a calming atmosphere. It was official. Classes started to fill.

Yoga was increasingly well received by the community and Christine wanted to plan for the future. She approached the economic development arm of the government of Nunavut for financial support for the next phase: yoga teacher training, a bigger porch, and more yoga equipment. The answer was "Yes," and Christine launched the first teacher training in Nunavut in 2017, preparing teachers to take yoga into the community.

Christine set up classes for the women's shelter, schools, and adults with disabilities. Christine was selected as a Governor General Leadership candidate, attending and co-chairing the Nunavut Study Tour to advocate for yoga and wellness in Nunavut.

It could be said that things are forever changed in our great white north, thanks to this remarkable woman who came in the most magical package—a young girl with moxie breakdancing on the streets of Ottawa.

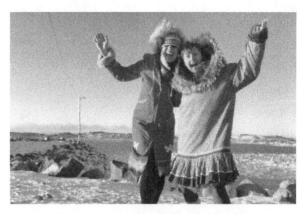

Kerry Lawson with Saimavik founder
Christine Lamothe

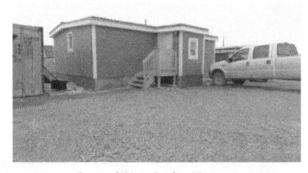

Saimavik Yoga Studio, Nunavut

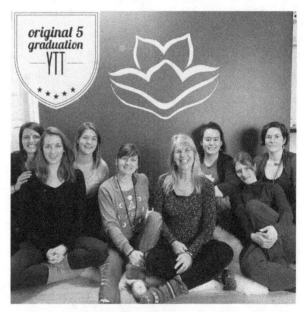

First teacher graduates, Nunavut, L to R: Danielle Samson, Erika Zell, Chantelle Masson, Christine Lamothe, Kerry Lawson, Gayle Kabloona, Sarah Scott & Carine Chalut

Kerry Lawson

Born London, Ontario, 1958 –

Kerry Lawson trains teachers at her four-acre ashram in Tusket, Nova Scotia, and is the first yoga therapist for the territory of Nunuvat. She takes groups to India and has appeared in the acclaimed Canadian film, Planet Yoga.

Kerry's mother, Martha Schmitz, was a yoga teacher in London, Ontario—she had learned from Kareen Zebroff's books and TV series in the 1960s. Kerry did not think it odd that her mother would sometimes take her out of school to help her with yoga classes for the physically challenged at the local YMCA. In those years, when it wasn't confused with the new health food yogurt, yoga was considered something that kooks and oddballs did. But to this mother-daughter team, it was as natural as breathing. They were both sensitive to other people's pain, (what we call "empaths" today) and had a strong desire to help. Kerry went on to become a full-time yoga teacher, studio owner, teacher trainer, and one of Canada's earliest yoga therapists. She has been successful in all of these, in large part, because she can tune in energetically with people and "feel their feelings."

As founder of Yoga with Kerry, run from her heritage home in Tusket, Nova Scotia, Kerry and her Indian-born husband, Kabir, conduct summer retreats called Living Yoga. These retreats are run in the style of an Indian ashram, complete with morning sun salutations, vegetarian food, classroom instruction, chanting, evening *satsang*, and the occasional Indian puja ceremony to mark a celebration. Their well-established teacher training program draws from their years of experience studying with Gopalakrishna and the well-known TKV Desikachar in India, and at Sivananda ashrams worldwide. To enable others to experience yoga in its motherland, Kerry and Kabir have taken over thirteen groups on pilgrimages to India.

With her reputation as a trainer, it was a natural fit that Kerry would team up with Christine Lamothe—owner of the Samaivik Studio in Iqaluit—to launch the first teacher training program in Nunavut and to set up classes in the schools. At the request of elders and the school board, Kerry conducted an hour-long class with a grade four Inuk girl. Says Kerry: "When we got to what was, for her, a difficult pose, we worked together quietly and meditatively and the elation on her face was very evident when she 'got it.' The elders saw that it was gentle and also esteem-building. The elders claim a similar practice in their culture goes back as long as India's. They said the meditative and quiet part resembled what they had to learn in order to sit for hours while ice fishing and hunting."

Kerry became an advisor to Nunavut schools on yoga and meditation programs for special groups, including those with trauma, histories of sexual abuse, and addictions. She flies to many small towns and outposts along with a translator of the Inuktitut language. "I love the north, my people there, and the work that has been done. Though sometimes challenging, it feels like it is the main purpose of being born to a yoga mom and 'falling' on that path of yoga."

Kerry's daughter, Natalie, in turn grew up in a yoga household. When entering school in the 1990s, Natalie found the school environment difficult to adapt to and more aggressive and competitive than her early home environment, so Kerry stepped in to offer yoga to the school. It was well received and after working with the school board and affiliates, yoga eventually became part of the Nova Scotia school curriculum. Natalie became certified as a yoga teacher and teaches in Squamish, British Columbia, completing the family wheel of three generations of teachers.

Kerry is expanding her yoga therapy trainings across Canada, encouraging Canadian teachers to organize themselves professionally and be confidant in their calling. She is part of the new world order that believes teaching skills of peace, stillness and equanimity in our education system makes the difference.

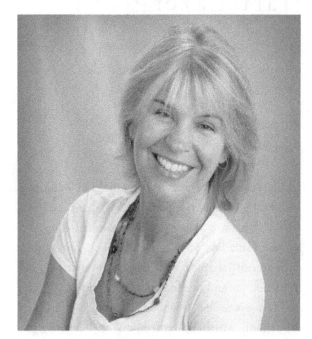

Kerry Lawson, Tusket, Nova Scotia

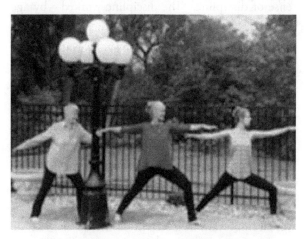

three generations of teachers: Martha Schwartz, Kerry Lawson, Natalie MacLeod

Hart Lazer

Born Winnipeg, Manitoba, 1953 –

Hart came from humble beginnings in Winnipeg. He became a trainer of yoga teachers par excellence, across Canada and on the international stage. He led the Canadian yoga movement and brought his entrepreneurial spirit to a profession that was still in its infancy and needed bold leadership.

Hart spent his boyhood in a Jewish rabbinical school, which he remembers as: "kindling my interest in spirituality and instilling in me a strong sense of discipline." The discipline worked—by age nineteen, Hart was a tennis pro. When he happened upon a yoga book written by Swami Sivananda, he likened the poses to the controlled body movements he felt in sports and was intrigued to know more.

In the 1970s, he met Swami Radha of the Sivananda tradition at a workshop and something was ignited. When he asked for a leave of absence from his job as a mental health counsellor in order to study at her ashram in Kootenay Bay, British Columbia, he was refused. He was very clear this was an important next step in his life, so in 1982, he resigned from his position and lived and studied at the ashram for six weeks.

Returning to Winnipeg, Hart took yoga classes at a synagogue with teacher Sheri Berkowitz, who encouraged him to study with well-known American Iyengar-trained teacher Ramanand Patel. He did, and it became a fruitful, long-term professional relationship. Now a senior teacher, Hart became co-owner of Yoga Centre Winnipeg as well as co-owner of Yoga Central Studio in Saskatoon.

Hart was involved in the early stages of the Iyengar community as they formed a Canadian teacher's organization. Says Hart of those times: "There was discussion about whether to go along with a teacher certification process or not. The decision was to have only one level so that there would be no hierarchy. Leaders Maureen and Bruce Carruthers felt strongly about this. The Canadian community decided to go along with it if it was one level and non-hierarchal. When I went to training at the Iyengar Institute in Pune, India, however, nothing was furthered. Some continued to push for multi-level certification and it was eventually passed. While in Pune, I witnessed an abusive situation between Mr. Iyengar and a student. I noticed I was enjoying the way he humiliated this person under the guise of ego breaking and I felt disgusted with myself for this reaction. I left as a result. There was a lack of trainers at the time and I decided to move forward on my own."

Further to trainings with Sheri and Ramanand, Hart studied the Ashtanga yoga system in depth with American David Swenson. He now found his stride and stepped in to fill the growing demand for teachers previously filled by senior visiting Americans.

When Hart was invited to speak and teach at the Ontario Yoga Teachers Association in the 1990's, he started off with the words, "Don't quit your day job," which raised a few eyebrows. Hart was making the point that his journey from teaching at seven dollars per class to his current US$2,000 per day was a road of hard work and commitment—plus good old-fashioned discipline. Today, his trainings run in China, Taiwan, Istanbul, Thailand, Japan, Berlin, and Cambodia, where he has a second studio. They usually run full with a wait list and he has up to five assistants.

In 2011, Hart made Montreal his home base and became part owner of United Yoga Montreal. His skills as a counsellor bring sensitivity and life experience into the classroom, allowing for a multi-dimensional exchange in his trainings. True to his own pioneer spirit, he encourages trainees to be confident and step up to opportunity as it is presented.

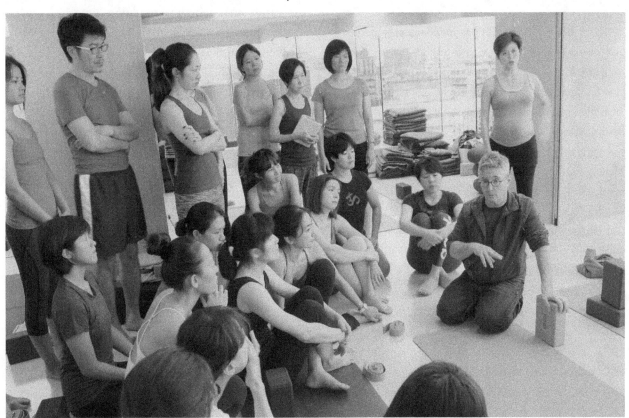

Hart Lazer teaching, Taipei, Taiwan

Sister Elaine MacInnes

Born Moncton, New Brunswick, 1924 –

Sister Elaine MacInnes has led a remarkable life. She was the first Canadian to found an organization to bring yoga and meditation into prisons in Eastern Canada and first Zen master nun in Canada.

Elaine was born to a musical family in New Brunswick. When her fiancé died in World War II, she went off to study music at The Julliard School in New York. From there she became a classical violinist for the Calgary and Edmonton symphonies.

She became a Roman Catholic nun in 1953. "I was thirty and for a Catholic person to choose a life work that is meaningful, it meant entering religious life and working in service for the rest of your life."

She went as a missionary to Japan, where she initially learned meditation to fit in. She stayed fifteen years, eventually becoming a Zen master. In 1976, she opened a meditation centre in Manila, Philippines, and taught meditation to political prisoners, some of whom had been tortured while in detention under Ferdinand Marcos's regime. This affected Sister Elaine deeply and she became a strong advocate for restorative justice, choosing prison work as her full-time vocation. Her work gained her international recognition and she was invited to England to be executive director of the Prison Phoenix Trust, based in Oxford. Launched in 1989, the PPT was an outgrowth of the Prison-Ashram Project, which was co-founded in 1973 by the American psychologist Ram Dass and yoga teacher Bo Lozoff. (Lozoff's book, *We're All Doing Time,* was the first yoga book written specifically for inmates.) The PPT gave inmates an alternative to doing time by viewing their confined small space as an ashram in which to practice simple postures and breath-centred meditation. Under Sister Elaine's directorship, the program flourished into a powerful project that improved prisoners' self-esteem and reduced prison violence.

Following her return home she was determined to introduce the program to Canada's prisons. She founded the Freeing the Human Spirit project in 2004. With a focus on the importance of yoga postures along with meditation, FHS collaborated with Yoga Outreach, a program involved with yoga in prisons in British Columbia. Initially, the FHS project faced a lot of resistance. Frequently challenged on meditation's doctrine or philosophy, Sister Elaine would respond, "I am not teaching a philosophy. I'm just doing something that requires no thought. It just takes time—and silence. The inner garbage gradually just disappears. There's no philosophy there at all. There's no philosophy in peace. In prison, as in a monastery or ashram, there is no waiting for this or that. Every minute is 'it.'" She called the prisons one by one to sell them on the benefits to prisoners and worked tirelessly to obtain the funding needed for a purpose some felt was frivolous.

Bearing fruit, the program eventually had fifty-two volunteers in twenty Canadian institutions. Sister Elaine's work opened doors to successfully educate prison staff on yoga and meditation and pave the way for teachers to enter. It won her the Order of Canada in 2011.

Sister Elaine retired in 2013, and passed her program on to the John Howard Society of Canada. She was featured in a documentary called "The Fires That Burn," by Vision TV and is the author of six books. Although a trailblazer and a legend, she does not see herself that way. As she wrote in the forward to her book, *Light Sitting in Light*, "I am extraordinarily ordinary."

She resides in Our Lady's Missionaries convent in Toronto. Says Elaine as she approaches her ninety-fifth birthday: "The older I get, the more complete I feel. I am still understanding myself and I am still becoming. I am impatient with my body now, though, but it is behaving normally and it is bowing out."

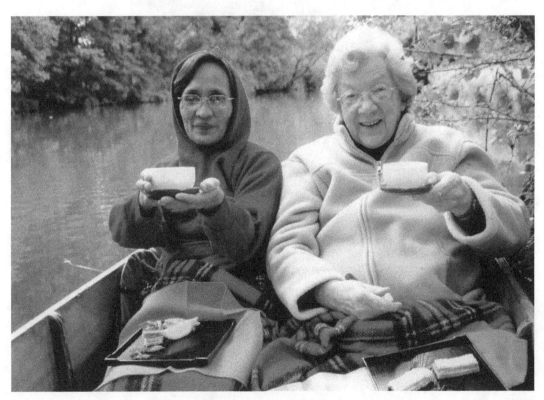

Sr. Rosario Battung and Sr. Elaine MacInnes, *Scarb*oro Missions Magazine

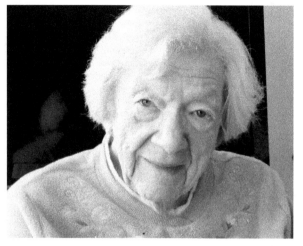

Elaine McInnes, founder, FTHS

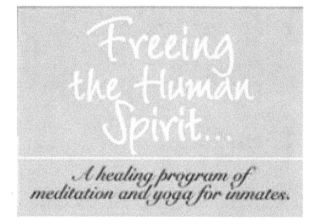

Freeing the Human Spirit, FTHS

Donna Martin

Born Prince Albert, Saskatchewan, 1947 –

Donna is credited with being a pioneer in teaching yoga as psychotherapy to mental health professionals at a time when the subject was little understood.

Donna's fascination with yoga started in the late 1960s. She bought books by Richard Hittleman and Indra Devi and began practicing while earning her BA and teaching degree at Western University in London, Ontario.

Moving to Kamloops, British Columbia, in 1974, Donna took a workshop at the YWCA with a visiting teacher. When she was approached by the Y program director to teach yoga classes, Donna asked, "Why me? " to which the director replied, "Because you are the only person in the workshop who can do a headstand!" Thus began her yoga teaching career. Donna opened the first yoga studio in Kamloops, which she ran successfully for ten years. Her TV show, called "Yoga for You," ran on the local community cable channel. She was frequently surprised when people recognized her in other provinces, only to discover later that the cable show was sometimes sold to other cities.

Donna was not content with just teaching yoga as a physical practice. She had a natural curiosity about how asana practice could reveal our beliefs and personalities. She knew that approaching practice with a meditative mind was revealing, but was there more? She got intrigued about a somatic psychotherapy system called Hakomi, which originated with Ron Kurtz of Oregon in the late 1970s, and she worked closely with Kurtz for twenty years until his death in 2011. She saw how the Hakomi method was mindfulness meditation based, although there was little awareness of mindfulness at the time. It was known as a method to reveal "core material" composed of emotional memories and deeply held beliefs, and Donna saw its compatibility with yoga, and she brought it into her classrooms. She encouraged partner work where one person would help the other to become aware of embodied habits. To process core material by witnessing asana and breath practice was groundbreaking work for its time and it led Donna to establish her own system, called Psoma Therapy.

As a full-time yoga teacher, Donna realized that the greatest benefit her students received from yoga and meditation was stress management. She also realized that the true source of stress is the way we react to life and organize our experiences; we often use coping strategies such as substance abuse, which in turn cause more stress and suffering. When Donna worked as a counsellor in the 1990s at the Phoenix Centre in Kamloops, she introduced her Psoma Therapy techniques to help clients interrupt the addiction cycle. She began to publish books and articles, becoming a stress-management consultant and educator.

When the practice of mindfulness meditation started to gain momentum around 2000, Donna was already leading edge. Her trainings appealed to addiction counsellors, psychologists, and mental health professionals interested in the renaissance of the field of body psychotherapy to assist their clients.

Professional groups began to host Donna internationally in the US (including Hawaii), Japan, Europe, Indonesia, South America, Argentina, and Mexico. Donna's trainings help others let go of judgment and unnecessary "efforting" in order to access inherent joy. She is a testament to her work because of her ever-present, trademark smile—she is seldom seen without it and it is genuine. It is part of her huge appeal and it invites everyone around her to drop into joy right along with her.

Says Donna of her lifetime work: "There is a subtle but important difference between Psoma yoga and other approaches. It focuses on the importance of curiosity and self-discovery versus trying to force change to happen. It is a process of getting people curious rather than judgmental in how they view themselves and this in itself is a huge paradigm shift." She adds, "The way we practice yoga is the way we live our life—if our practice is filled with a sense of wonder, mindful awareness, gratitude, compassion, and loving presence, this will inform and transform the way we live."

Donna now calls British Columbia's South Okanagan home. She still travels globally, training

professionals. Despite her busy schedule, she continues as a long-time presenter at Hollyhock on Cortes Island and the Hui Ho'olana retreat center on the island of Molokai, Hawaii.

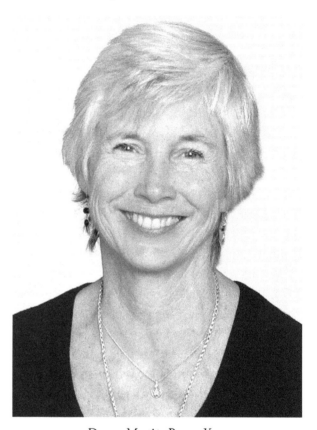

Donna Martin, Psoma Yoga

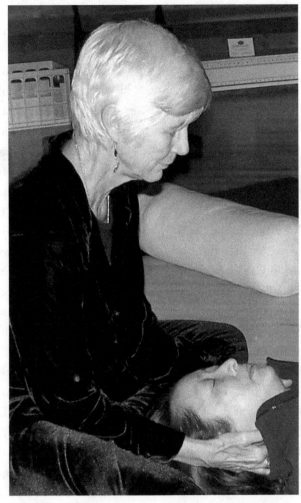

Donna Martin teaching Hollyhock, Cortes Island

Marlene Mawhinney

Born Toronto, Ontario, 1938 –

Marlene Mawhinney specializes in teaching therapeutic yoga for special populations such as those with cardiac ailments, MS, asthma, cancer, and brain injury. She was chosen by yoga master BKS Iyengar for the first wave of certification in Canada and she started teaching in 1972—she is still teaching today at over eighty years young.

Marlene started yoga on TV with Kareen Zebroff in 1970, while recovering from an illness. It kindled her interest and she saw the possibility of yoga improving her health. She took her first class with Sivananda-style teacher Lila Ostermann at the newly opened Yoga Centre Toronto in the early 1970s. Lila impressed her with her charismatic nature and single-minded commitment. Although Marlene took classes in the 3HO and Kripalu styles of yoga as well, she stayed with the YCT and Sivananda method and eventually received teacher certification in that style in 1975. She then opened her own yoga studio in Newmarket, Ontario. It was through Esther Myers in Toronto in the late 1970s that she was introduced to Iyengar-style yoga; a spark was ignited that that was to open up a pathway for life and became her style of

choice. When she closed her studio to become more involved in the larger community of YCT she started to teach Iyengar yoga classes there in 1983. In 1986, Marlene became president of the board of directors of YCT and she still holds that role today.

Marlene became a founding member of the Iyengar Yoga Association of Canada. She took her first trip to Pune, India, in 1985 to study with Mr. Iyengar personally. Here at the Ramamani Institute, she was greatly influenced by the man she came to respectfully refer to as "Guruji." She dedicated herself to Iyengar methodology and returned to the institute and intensive trainings on seventeen different occasions. She particularly appreciated his refinement of asana to therapeutic poses that involved intelligent use of props, correct sequencing, and long, timed holds. Says Marlene: "I appreciated his commitment and dedication of his life to his art. His work had an authenticity and integrity that spoke to me."

Marlene spent many years teaching up to twenty classes per week at YCT. Like the master who taught her, she kept a keen eye on her students, observing their progress firsthand. Change in skin colour, a slight shift in breathing—all were part of the subtleties of her training. As a testament to her consistent hard work, she is recognized internationally for her expertise in writing yoga programs for health challenges. She has written the *40-Day Sadhana Manual*, and two volumes of *Iyengar Yoga Practices*.

The YCT under Marlene's guidance is the only Iyengar studio in Canada to conduct cardiac classes, MS classes, classes in yoga to overcome pain, brain injury classes, and recovery classes for cancer, asthma, and other immune issues. In these classes, Marlene supervises a team of assistants made up of teachers and teacher trainees.

Says Marlene: "My special needs classes are my personal interest and passion, evolved out of the twenty-seven years I was in Pune, working directly under Mr. Iyengar's guidance. The therapeutic form stems from an asana being adapted to the individual's needs and specific ailment. In his book *Light on Life*, Mr. Iyengar says pain is a privilege and that it is out of pain and personal illness that we learn. That is his teaching and indeed that has been my learning."

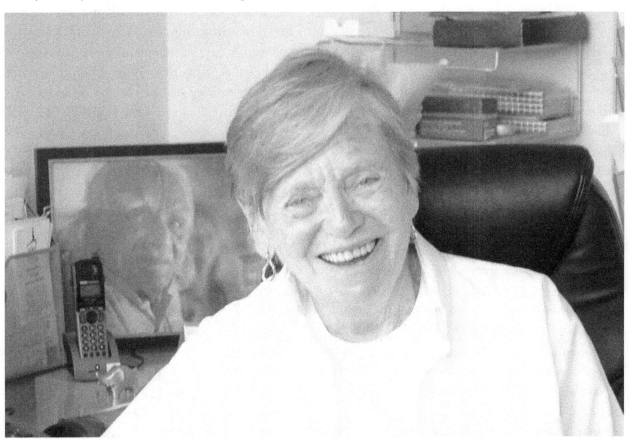

Marlene Mawhinney, Toronto, Ontario, 2019

Jody Myers

Born Halifax, Nova Scotia, 1951 –

Jody is one of those people you expect to meet when you go to the Maritimes. Earthy and ultra-friendly, she knows everyone and wants you to meet them.

She's also a driving force behind organizing yoga in Nova Scotia for the last thirty years.

Her interest started when she attended the first yoga centre in Halifax, in the late 1970s, called Kripalu Yoga Society. She followed up by training at the early Kripalu Center in Summit Station, Pennsylvania, in 1980. Here, she met Swami Kripalvananda of India, for whom the ashram was named after. In her words, "I received 'diksha,' the Guru's blessing of grace, which led to a profound mystical experience. It is hard to put into words—it was a beautiful, elevated feeling. I wanted to live my life with love and service, there was no doubt."

Jody went to the ashram a physical education teacher and returned to Halifax a devoted yogi. Upon her return, she formed her own yoga business and taught weekly classes at hospitals, the university, government offices, and schools. She returned for many trainings at Kripalu with Amrit Desai, whom she also hosted three times in Nova Scotia.

When a sex scandal hit Kripalu in 1994, resulting in the forced resignation of Amrit Desai, Jody has this to say, "I waited seven years out of respect for the residents at the Kripalu Center for them to work out differences with Amrit Desai. After that time, it was still a mess. One teacher said, 'People who want to heal their relationship with Gurudev will have to go and work it out with him in person.' A lot of people did just that. I felt that my guru had made some really big mistakes, but he was still my guru. After those seven years were over, I went back and took Amrit's new teacher program at a new location and it was well worth it. I always felt that I had my own personal karma with Amrit Desai and it had little to do with events at the Kripalu Centre. After that seven-year period, I just wanted to get on with life."

She did that by founding a Teacher Training program in the Maritimes in 2000, naming it Atlantic Yoga Teacher Training. It was to prove a year of trusting in her own gifts going forward. Partly to celebrate her newfound independence, she organized a millennium celebration at Dalhousie University in Halifax to bring together the various yoga communities. Over 100 people registered.

Although over the years Jody added several other styles of yoga to her training—Bikram, Iyengar, Art of Living, Asthanga Power Yoga, and Anasura—she remains committed to the Kripalu Meditation in Motion approach.

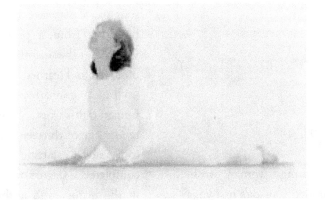

Jody Myers, Halifax, Nova Scotia, 1966

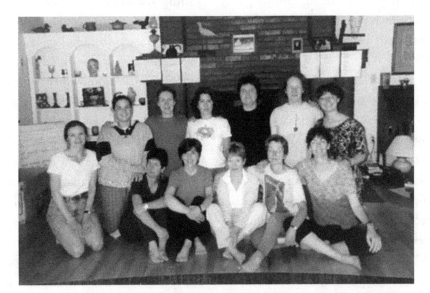

Atlantic Yoga Teacher Graduates,
(first row L to R) Chris MacDonald, Helen Slade, Kerry Oliver,
Sonya Breeze Isha Ward, Jody Myers
(back row L to R) Stephanie Laidlaw, Ilene Orr, Bonnie Vanechuck, Jean Short,
Gail Salsbury, Karen Hollett

Jessica Robertson

Born Claremont, Ontario, 1977 –

Jessica Robertson, a young woman from Claremont, Ontario, co-founded Canada's first yoga studio chain in 2004. Modo (previously Moksha) studios grew from Jessica attending Ashtanga Fellowship yoga camps each year as a child with her parents. It was here she met Baba Hari Dass and his lessons shaped her life.

Baba Hari Dass was a silent monk from 1952 until his death in 2018. He was a well-known Indian mystic, brought to the attention of the West by Harvard psychology professor Richard Alpert (Ram Dass) in his popular 1971 book, *Be Here Now*. Baba Hari Dass was known for expounding simple teachings by writing on a chalkboard that he wore on a rope around his neck. He became a powerful influence in Jessica's parent's lives, and, in turn, in Jessica's life as well. Says Jessica: "This man taught me, by example, the meaning of compassion, simplicity and integrity and joy."

Jessica's parents taught her the value of having a daily *sadhana* (spiritual practice) and the importance of applying yogic principles to everyday life situations. They were effective activists, dedicating years of their life to a forum called *Land over Landing* that sought to preserve agricultural lands and historic buildings from a proposed airport in Pickering, Ontario. (The dispute is still continuing.) Jessica observed and learned.

Jessica gravitated toward environmental and human rights work. She began public speaking at the tender age of thirteen for Amnesty International on topics such as starting community-based groups. She completed a degree at McGill University, majoring in the history and anthropology of medicine and Russian literature. While at McGill, she worked with Earthsave, a Vancouver-based non-profit group promoting environmentally friendly food choices. She worked in Panama for Panama National Federation of Parents of Children with Disability, a program that promoted education for children with developmental disabilities. She also learned how to speak Spanish.

When she met like-minded activist Ted Grand, it was a colliding of ideals in the most impactful way. They saw how their mutual commitment to personal evolution through yoga as well as their ingrained sense of planetary responsibility could translate to running yoga studios with a difference, and Moksha Yoga was founded in 2004. Today there are over sixty-three studios, now named Modo Yoga, across Canada, and over fifteen in the United States as well as studios in Paris, Sydney, and Geneva. Many admirers emulate their concept and it is closely watched by skeptics because it is quite, well, radical.

As Canada's first and largest yoga franchise-type chain, the Modo business plan has been one of carefully monitored growth. Sensitive to pressures from the marketplace to keep pace with a rapidly growing industry, they have resisted growth that will compromise their shared values. They follow a stringent screening process for new studio owners who must agree with their policies of environmentally friendly building products, community fundraising projects, and, obviously, a dedication to being a skilled yoga teacher.

Others are taking cues from this dynamic model of harmonizing business and social responsibility. Through their example, Jessica and Ted invite thoughtful responses to such issues as protecting nature and providing financial assistance to those less fortunate, all while leading a thriving business entity.

Jessica Robertson is home-based in Costa Rica, while travelling regularly across the US and Canada to train teachers and teams for the Modo Yoga network. She visits Claremont, Ontario regularly to see her parents who chuckle that they are still "self-proclaimed hippies" who continue to follow the teachings of Baba Hari Dass and live a simple yoga lifestyle.

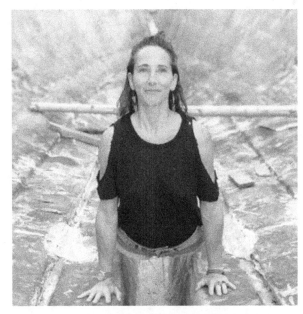

Jessica Robertson, co-founder, Moda (Moksha) Yoga. Photo: Florian Kluster

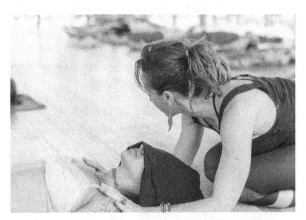

Jessica Robertson teaching, photo by Florian Kluster

Rose Rosenstone

Born Sydney, Australia, 1910; died Montreal, Quebec, 2002

When Australian-born Rose met and married a Canadian in 1935, she relocated to his birthplace of Montreal. Once they settled, they opened a restaurant, which they ran for many years. Rose continued to run it even after her husband died in 1965.

Rose had a keen interest in mysticism, spirituality, and healing. She possessed a strong desire to help those less fortunate—particularly youth. This was, in part, influenced by her early years witnessing her father suffer from depression. He once attempted suicide by jumping off South Heads in Sydney, Australia, only to be rescued by a passerby who jumped into the water after him. The experience left a deep impression on Rose, opening her up to acts of compassion.

Rose was to become the first Sivananda-style yoga teacher in Canada, but her path was somewhat circuitous. She began with philanthropic work, founding the Montreal Forward House in 1957—a non-profit organization providing residential programs for those with mental illness. She was also an active member of the Pythian Sisters, a fraternal order that performed charitable works at places such as the Douglas Mental Hospital in Verdun, Quebec.

Rose was continuously seeking spirituality and healing. Although yoga knowledge was scanty at the time, she had picked up Swami Vishnudevananda's voluminous book, The Illustrated Book of Yoga, and dug in. When she went to hear him lecture at his newly established Sivananda Centre on Boulevard St. Lawrence in 1961, she was enraptured by his message and it became a turning point for her. She saw the depth of yoga as a healing modality that could help the populations she worked with. She became a passionate student and part of Swami Vishnudevanda's inner circle, which helped him establish roots in his new home of Canada. In turn, in 1962, the swami chose Rose as his first teacher in Canada. Certificates were not yet given out, but that was not of importance to Rose. She had found her path. Little did she know that she was the first of what would be thousands of teachers trained by Swami Vishnudevananda in the ensuing years and that his prolific work would expand internationally. Marilyn Rossner soon followed Rose as a Sivananda yoga teacher. The two shared a close friendship that lasted their lifetimes, forged by their mutual desire to help those with special needs. They became renowned not only for their humanitarian work, but their colourful dress, which often included animal prints, hats, and beads, reflecting the rebelliousness of the 1960s and '70s.

Rose's granddaughter, Heather Silberberg, was born in 1977 and absorbed yoga from her grandmother as a natural part of daily life. She recalls coming downstairs in the morning and seeing her granny standing on her head and joining in. In 1995, Rose moved to Vancouver to be with her family. Says Heather: "She would give me private sessions sitting in her chair with her cane. I never did have to learn in a studio. It wasn't just the asanas—I learned breath and meditation and how to use stillness to drop into a peaceful centre. I taught yoga to my fellow travellers while backpacking in Europe and at my various places of work. My grandmother read and lived by the philosophy of yoga—that we can't be peaceful warriors until we achieve inner peace through diligent practice. Behind my grandmother's outrageous sense of humour was a serious, purpose-led life. It taught me, in turn, to live my life meaningfully, even when I found myself in challenging corporate roles. It is still my greatest thrill to teach and see the awakening in others; it is such a worthwhile path." Today, Heather works at the Down Syndrome Society in Vancouver and teaches at Open Door Yoga Studios. She formalized her training by receiving a teacher's certificate at Sivananda Centre Val Morin in 2010, forty-eight years after her grandmother had earned hers.

Rose was actively teaching yoga and leading spiritual circles in Vancouver until age eighty-five; she passed peacefully at age ninety.

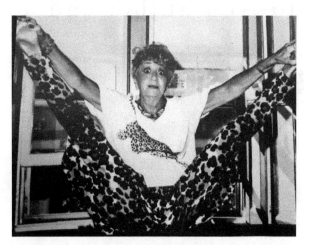

Rose Rosenstone at age 80, first Sivananda teacher

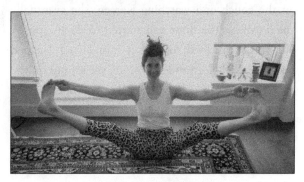

Rose's granddaughter Heather Silberberg, 2019

Jo-Ann Sutherland

Born Fort Francis, Ontario, 1944 –

While living in Montreal in 1970, Jo-Ann started yoga on TV with Kareen Zebroff, like so many others of her era. Jo-Ann had back issues and chronic bronchitis. Though she started by sitting on the couch and watching Kareen, she eventually got down on the floor and started to do the poses. She was astonished to find it immediately helped her backache. Keen to learn more, she set out on the path that led to her being a teacher and opening the first yoga studio in Saskatchewan many years later.

Jo-Ann found a teacher at a community centre in Roxboro, Montreal, where she stayed for two years studying the Sivananda method.

In 1975, she moved to Edmonton and enrolled in classes. "It was during this time that I really got hooked," Jo-Ann says. "I also credit my daily practice with helping me keep mentally and physically strong during a painful divorce."

She later lived in Winnipeg for four years and studied with Iyengar-style teacher Sheri Berkowitz, and she began to teach there. Jo-Ann remarried in 1984 and moved her home to Saskatoon. She started teaching classes at the University of Saskatchewan and the YWCA while working a day job at the potash mine.

Jo-Ann opened Saskatchewan's first yoga studio on 7th Avenue in Saskatoon. It was a small studio, fitting only ten people; the year was 1990, and if Saskatoon wasn't ready, she was going to make it ready.

As classes grew, she quit her day job at the mine and opened a new studio at a bigger location. She stayed here for the next twenty-four years, introducing thousands of people to yoga. Her instructional DVDs, her TV program, "Yoga for the Inside Out," and her weekly magazine columns were popular, and she gained a province-wide reputation as a demanding but caring, teacher. In 1998, she became one of the first level teachers to receive an Iyengar certificate in Canada. As part of her certification, Jo-Ann was required to go to India regularly to study at the Iyengar institute in Pune, which she did five times. Jo-Ann often hosted annual meetings for the Canadian Iyengar Yoga Association, who considered Saskatoon a halfway point for people to meet from across the country.

Although retired and still living in Saskatoon, Jo-Ann teaches chair yoga at the Apache Yoga Center in Arizona, where she goes as a "snowbird." She gives her time generously to others who have health issues, teaching them how to use yoga for relief of symptoms.

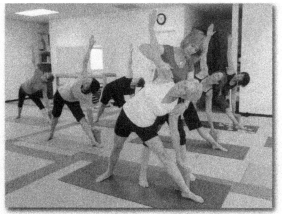

Jo-Ann Sutherland, founder of JNS Yoga Studio, not only teaches yoga students, she also instructs and certifies Iyengar yoga teachers. (Photo: Jeff Lyons/StarPhoenix)

Yoga flourishing in Saskatoon

by Jeannie Armstrong
SP Creative Features Editor

It's a yoga revolution.

According to Yoga Directory Canada, over 1.5 million Canadians practice one form of yoga or another. Another 2.1 million Canadians say they intend to try yoga within the next 12 months, according to the Print Measurement Bureau.

Why is yoga soaring in popularity? Many see yoga as a path to improved well-being, says Jo-Ann Sutherland, a nationally certified instructor with the Iyengar Yoga Association of Canada and owner of JNS Yoga Studio, located at 96 – 33rd Street East in Saskatoon.

Sutherland is considered one of Western Canada's foremost yoga authorities. She began taking yoga 39 years ago in Montreal as a means to improve her own health. She progressed from student to teacher seven years later, and started instructing classes in Winnipeg.

Sutherland relocated to Saskatoon in 1984, and began teaching yoga classes at the local Y. In 1990, she founded JNS Yoga Studio in Saskatoon.

"When I moved to Saskatoon,

there wasn't any yoga here. I was a yogi before yoga was cool," chuckles Sutherland.

Sutherland not only teaches yoga students, she also instructs and certifies Iyengar yoga teachers.

In 1985, Sutherland began studying the Iyengar Method of Yoga, developed by renowned yoga master B.K.S. Iyengar. She gained national certification in the Iyengar system, and now is involved in training and certifying other instructors.

Sutherland has travelled to Pune, India many times for continued instruction at the yoga institute founded by B.K.S. Iyengar 35 years ago. At age 92, he still remains actively involved with the institute.

"Iyengar yoga is more aligned. It's about getting the body and the mind aligned. Iyengar yoga has many therapeutic benefits," says Sutherland.

"Mr. Iyengar recognized that all bodies are different, with unique strengths and weaknesses. To accommodate these differences, he developed a variety of props, including wooden blocks, chairs, blankets and

(Continued on Page 6)

IN BALANCE 5

Jo-Ann Sutherland opens Saskatoon's first studio, 1990

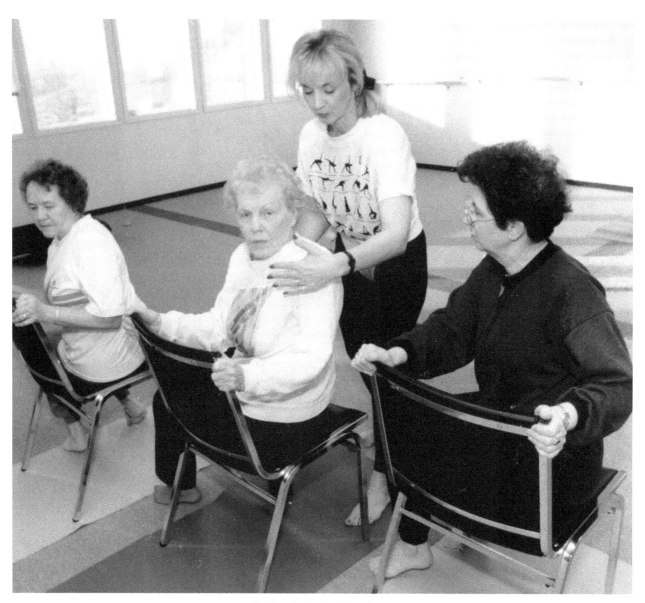

Jo-Ann Sutherland teaching

Bev Zizzy

Born Canora, Saskatchewan, 1953 –

Bev was the founding president of the Yoga Association of Saskatchewan, an association created in 1976 by the first Regina yoga teachers to provide a basis for professional development. As a language teacher, singer/songwriter, and recording artist, Bev attributes much of her inspiration to over forty years of yoga practice. Says Bev: "Every challenge, every accomplishment, every hill, every valley, every breath I take, every song I have written, every song I sing—all have been influenced by the practice of yoga I have been devoted to for over four decades, and its fundamental values that have shaped my life, all of which are reflected in my music."

Bev moved to Regina in 1967 and, in 1971, while an undergraduate student at the University of Regina, she began her study of yoga with early Regina teacher Elisabeth Smith. In her role as the founding president of YAS, Bev helped host many senior teachers from both sides of the border: Marcia Moore, Donald Moyer, Ramanand Patel Patel, Judith Lasater, Shirley French, Shirley Johannesen, and others who helped build the yoga scene in Regina. Never a woman of half measures, Bev threw herself into each influence of the time—Sivananda, Iyengar, and Ashtanga styles—eventually returning to her classic Sivananda roots.

Her ongoing yoga practice energized her thirty-five-year career as a language and literature teacher, first in Northern Saskatchewan, and then Regina. This same dedication to daily yoga practice also fuelled her creativity as a recording artist, which she began while still teaching full-time, with her first EP release, "If My Life Were a Song," in 2002.

When Bev lost her only daughter in a car accident at age eighteen, she credits her yoga practice with giving her the resilience to carry on, in addition to the support of her community of family, friends, and students. She channeled the raw emotion of this loss into her music, and the result was a soulful and stirring album, *Woman in Black* (2009), followed by her second commercial album release, *Standing on a Platform of Kindness* (2016).

Her catharsis through yoga and music deepened her compassion and desire to help others. Bev describes herself as "a lifelong yogi committed to the power of giving." Her global philanthropic activities have included raising funds for AIDS relief, as well as numerous foster children and girls' education sponsorships. She is a recipient of the Regina YWCA's Women of Distinction Award.

One of Bev's favourite quotes is from the Buddha: "If you knew what I know about the power of giving, you would not let a single meal pass without sharing it in some way."

Bev still calls Regina home, though she spends winters in Thailand and Bali, where she practices Ashtanga yoga. Her yoga practice continues to evolve as she currently studies a form of tantric yoga reminiscent of Andre Van Lysebeth's classic text, *Yoga Self Taught* (1968). She finds it astounding to have come right back to where she started after a lifetime of diverse yoga teachings. She now embraces a meditative, energy-based traditional Sivananda style. For her, it provides testimony that the practice of yoga is not a static entity, but a personal process.

Bev hosts a travel blog on spiritual and sacred spaces around the world. She continues to attract crowds to her at the drop of a hat—and reach for her guitar—but she is never far from her beloved yoga mat.

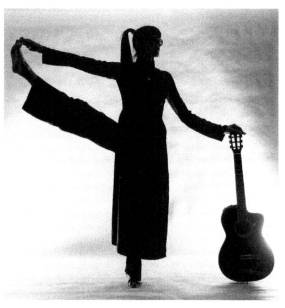

Bev Zizzy records "Still Standing"

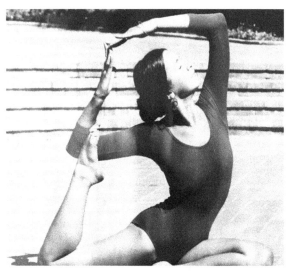

Bev Zizzy in Raja, Kapotanasana, 1971

Part 4
Swamis

I call this group of pioneers the Swamis, but they could also be called monks or gurus. Swamis are often misconstrued. For those old enough to remember early comic books, the term conjures up images of an Indian wearing a white head turban, beset with jewels, who can perform magic. I remember Swami Radha joking once about whether people came to her ashram as serious students "or just out of curiosity to see a real live swami." Although the *siddhas* (special powers) of a swami are real, they are rare and found only in the true masters. Swamis are ordinary people like you and me who, at some point in their lives, have a burning desire for self-realization. To do this and succeed, they embark on a spiritual path, or *sadhana*, making it a priority. They relinquish worldly pursuits, which are only distractions. In other words, they adopt a lifestyle that supports their inner quest. Their spiritual practice is to strive for mastery over one's smaller self of habit patterns, roles, and identifications so that the eternal Self may be directly experienced—a tall order! Swamis take their vows, called an initiation, with a chosen tradition that is passed from guru to guru. They become part of a metaphysical chain, as it were, called a lineage. Selflessness and service to others defines them, which they believe creates the right karma. Swamis or gurus attract a lot of followers, or students, who they are happy to help but whom they would prefer find their own spiritual footing and not make gods of them. In fact, they would be happy to be viewed as fellow aspirants on the path rather than as guru and disciple. Students often set their guru up for failure by forgetting they are simply human and that they are also aspirants.

The swamis featured in this book were the first swamis in Canada. None of them were born in Canada, but they adopted Canada as their country. It just so happened they were all initiated into the same lineage, although at different times and places. These swamis spent time daily in meditation and silence, but they were also hard workers. We can learn a lot from these swamis. They displayed enviable skills at conducting a balanced life, something most people struggle with in today's world. If you judge them just by their selfless acts, they have been exemplary role models. It is my belief time will look back kindly on them as visionaries of peace. Here's a look at how three swamis with very different personalities followed their destinies in the (sometimes) wilds of Canada.

Swami Radha
(Sylvia Hellman)

Born Berlin, Germany, 1911; died Spokane, Washington, 1995

Sylvia Hellman broke the established norms of the time by becoming the first Western female initiate in a monastic order in the West at a time when most orders were traditionally male. When you think about that, it is really something.

She lit a path forward for women in a long-held patriarchal lineage, although it is unclear that was her intent. She was the first swami to reside in Canada and she became an inspiration for women of all faiths.

Her decision to come to Canada in selfless service to a divine mission seems to have been timely, given the tidal wave shift toward the feminine brought forward by yoga in the West. How did this come to be, and why Sylvia?

Sylvia grew up in Germany in a privileged family. She excelled as a dancer and photographer and had a bright future. Then World War II came, and with it, Sylvia experienced one tragedy after another. The Gestapo executed her husband, Wolfgang, for helping Jews escape. She lost both her parents in the war. She

managed to move on with her life only to lose her second husband, a composer and violinist named Albert Hellman, when he died in her arms from a stroke one year into their marriage. It devastated her to her core. This is when she reached a climactic stage of grief and, with it, an existential crisis. She questioned all existence. Was it only to suffer? Where was the meaning to it all?

Sylvia resisted brokenness and her experiences deepened her compassion for all human beings. She sensed a strong calling, although she had no spiritual context for it at the time. It was here she began a deep spiritual inquiry. With the war ended, she had a two-year transition as a housekeeper in England before she headed for Canada in 1951.

Like other yogis mentioned in this book, Sylvia sought a fresh start and a peaceful life in Canada to heal the scars of war. She settled in Montreal and carved out a living as a dance instructor and photographer. She began a meditation practice, following her now-familiar spiritual pull. It was here in a meditation that she vividly saw the face of Swami Sivananda Saraswati of India, even though she did not know who he was at that time.

But one day on a walk she saw his face on a book in a bookstore window and she immediately knew the identity of the face in her vision. She wrote him a letter and he invited her to his ashram in Rishikesh, India, telling her, "Come to me—we have known each other many lifetimes."

As founder of the internationally recognized Divine Light Society, Swami Sivananda was a much-revered master. Sylvia became his first Western female student and he gave her rigorous training. As meets tradition, he initiated her in the Saraswati order and gave her the name Swami Radha, which means "success" in Sanskrit.

Thus began the spiritual path of a woman who had refused to succumb to despair and was willing to live her life on faith.

She returned to Montreal in 1956 as a renunciate in orange robes, and she received a lot of attention! She began to speak publicly, showing films about her experiences in India and teaching yoga classes; CBC Radio and newspapers often interviewed her. She had been instructed by Sivananda to "abstain from all actions which arise from ambition and selfish desire and to give up mental and emotional attachment to life in this world." Thus, she learned to live with no money or employment, trusting her needs would be met. That same year, supporters in her Montreal group who were part of the India Canada Association, flew her to Vancouver to lecture on Indian philosophy.

Her first talk on yoga and reincarnation drew over 550 people, and was written up in the *Vancouver Sun* as "Woman Yogi Draws Big Crowd Here." Future talks were held at various Sikh temples. She continued to give talks in Vancouver, Victoria, and Toronto. Her topics were billed as: Spiritual Diary for Effective Living, Yoga as a Universal System, Yoga and Vedanta in the Modern World, and one cited yoga for "freedom from those habit masters, cigarettes and alcohol." The support she received made her choose to stay in Vancouver, where she started attracting a small number of committed

followers. One of the first was Joe Gnilke, a carpenter and jack-of-all-trades who was to play a large role over the next thirteen years in helping Swami Radha realize her dreams. They pooled money together to purchase and renovate a ten-room home in Burnaby as their first communal ashram, or spiritual hermitage. It was run similarly to an Indian ashram—daily devotions were *bhajans*, *kirtan*, and *satsang*. Joe was to accompany Swami Radha on a world pilgrimage where she lectured and toured—he kept her safe and rested and maintained diaries of their trip.

As the Burnaby ashram grew, they began looking for the "mountains and lakes" Swami Sivananda had said was her destiny for a permanent ashram. Joe, in particular, was keen that Radha's unrelenting determination would pay off. By now, Swami Radha reached all decisions in her life by Divine faith. She followed a series of introductions and coincidences until they found seventy-five acres of land in Kootenay Bay, British Columbia, oddly registered under the Sanskrit name *Yasodhara*, which was the name of the Buddha's wife.

The land was cleared and the ashram built by faithful Joe and many selfless people who shared a common goal—a spiritual community for others to come and study yoga and examine their lives. Yasodhara launched a three-month residential teacher training program in 1976, and although an isolated location, it began to attract international students. It is here that Swami Radha spent the rest of her life inspiring a community while writing for posterity until she died in 1995.

She wrote her first book, *Kundalini Yoga for the West,* in 1978, and it was considered groundbreaking for its time. It was followed by many other notable publications with Timeless Books. Her writings threading western psychology with eastern teachings contributed to a growing trend at the time. Her Divine Light Invocation, a powerful healing meditation, has become well known in Canadian yoga circles and is considered her signature piece. Throughout all her work a call to inquiry and a challenge to character resonates—such was the legacy of Swami Radha.

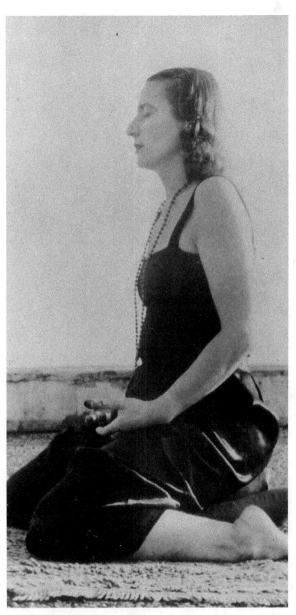

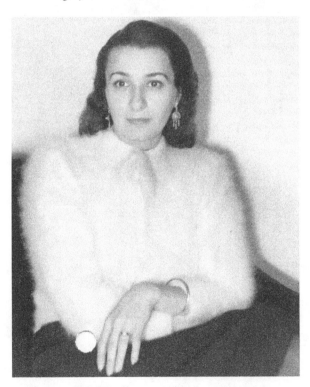

Sylvia Hellman, 1944, Germany

Sylvia Hellman meditating on a rooftop, Montreal, 1955

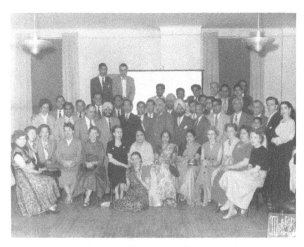

Montreal group, Swami Radha seated, 1956

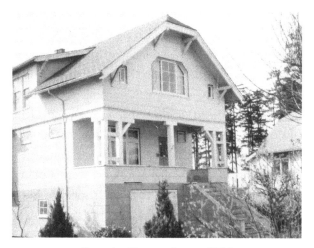

Burnaby House ashram, 1958

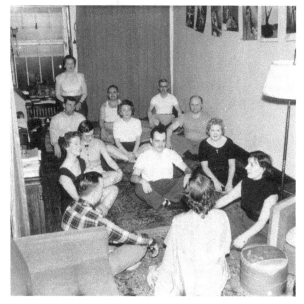

Swami Radha teaching in Montreal, 1956

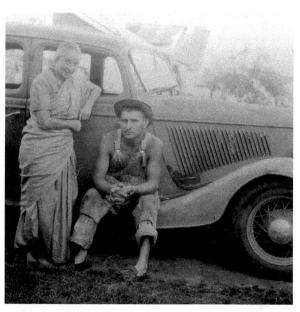

Swami Radha with Joe Gnilke, 1960

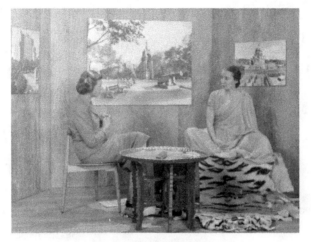

Swami Radha TV interview, Montreal

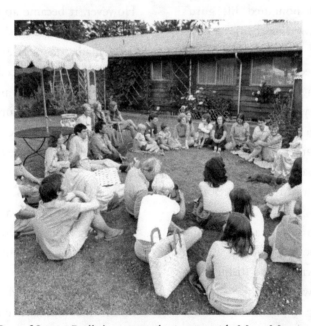

One of Swami Radha's many gatherings outside Many Mansions,
Yasodhara Ashram

Swami Vishnudevananda (Kuttan Nair)

Born Kerala, India, 1927; died Uttarakhand, India, 1993

Swami Vishnudevananda honoured his guru's request to take yoga teachings to the West. His life story resembles that of Swami Radha of the Kootenays—both were devotees of Swami Sivananda Saraswati of India and both became initiates into the Sivananda tradition. They can be credited with building the pillars of yoga in Canada—one opened an ashram in eastern Canada and the other in western Canada, both at about the same time. Despite the similar life purpose they each held, their personalities were very different.

Swami Vishnudevananda came across Swami Sivananda's writings while he was a young man in the Indian army. He felt drawn to go to Rishikesh to meet him. There, he took vows under the Sivananda Saraswati lineage, becoming a monk at the age of twenty.

He had a dedicated practice, mastering difficult, advanced hatha yoga techniques. When asked how he perfected ancient practices, he would say, "My Master touched me and opened my eye of intuition. All this knowledge returned to me from past lives." He went on to author *The Complete Illustrated Book of Yoga*, a voluminous book on hatha and raja yoga that gave him international recognition. He became famous for his quote "An ounce of practice is worth a ton of theory."

After ten years of living and studying under Swami Sivananda, he was told to spread the teachings of yoga to the West, with the words, "People are waiting." He taught all over North America, but he liked New York best and chose it as his home. However, it became apparent there were too many obstacles to his citizenship there. So, when his faithful Canadian supporters urged him to come back to Montreal and enticed him with premises to live and teach, he agreed, and in 1959 opened the first Sivananda Yoga Vedanta Centre in Montreal at Boulevard Saint-Laurent. Still open and thriving today, the centre is the site for countless Canadians' acknowledgement of their start in yoga, where they dropped in for classes or lectures.

Swami Vishnudevananda offered his visitors something more. In 1961, he launched the first yoga camp at a student's summer home. He took note of the fact that westerners were willing to go out into nature and give up all their material comforts to sleep on the floor and take cold showers. It seemed to him that building a camp with an austere, Indian ashram-style setting would succeed. In 1962, he launched a permanent yoga camp in the mountains near Val

Morin, Quebec. For this, Swami Vishnudevananda can be credited with originating the first yoga vacation. Here, he began a teacher training program that was the first of its kind in Canada. Many Canadian teachers owe their start to the trainings here. It could be said that the Sivananda style is the original in Canada, and it is impossible to measure the contribution it has made to Canadian communities.

Using the Val Morin Yoga Camp in Quebec as international headquarters, Swami Vishnudevananda went on to open nine other successful ashrams worldwide, which are credited with training over 45,000 teachers. This intercontinental weave of ashrams put Canada on the map as a yoga destination, attracting them to the uniqueness of Quebec and the beauty of the Laurentian Mountains, and the easy access from Montreal. His teachings comprised five principles: proper exercise, proper breathing, proper relaxation, proper diet (vegetarian), and meditation and positive thinking.

Perhaps Swami Vishnudevananda's most compelling legacy was his efforts for world peace. Disturbed by a vision he had of a world engulfed by flames from acts of war, he decided to act. He bought a plane and had it colourfully painted by the well-known artist Peter Max. He then went on peace flights over the world's trouble spots, starting with Belfast in Northern Ireland. A month later he flew to the Middle East on a peace flight over the Suez Canal during the Sinai War. Israeli military jets tried to force Swami Vishnudevananda to land, but he continued his mission unwaveringly. His message: "Man is free as a bird—overcome borders with flowers and love, not with guns and bombs." Accordingly, he glided over the Berlin Wall from West to East Germany in 1983 in an ultralight aircraft "armed" with two bouquets of marigolds and landed on a farm in Weissensee, East Germany. After being interrogated by East German authorities for four hours, he was put on the Metro with a cheese sandwich and sent back to West Berlin. Said the swami, "Symbolically, we want to show we cannot cross borders with guns, only with flowers. If they shoot me over the Berlin Wall, what difference is it? Many people have died for war; I shall die for peace."

Canadians were receptive to this message, the way being paved by the famous Give Peace a Chance bed-in with John Lennon and Yoko Ono in Montreal in 1969. Also coinciding at that time was the introduction of Transcendental Meditation® across Canada by Beatles' guru, Maharishi Mahesh Yogi.

By now an acclaimed, if slightly eccentric, Canadian peacemaker, Swami Vishnudevananda received further recognition when crowds gathered to watch him walk across hot coals in a cross-India tour in 1984—the pictures went worldwide. His message was that the human spirit can overcome "fire" of all kinds with single-minded focus.

Swami Vishnudevananda met with world spiritual leaders to promote interfaith dialogue. With help from lifelong devotee and visionary Marilyn Rossner, he organized yearly conferences on such topics as yoga and science, the frontiers of consciousness, sustainable living, and nuclear disarmament.

While on pilgrimage in India in 1993, Swami Vishnudevananda achieved *mahasamadhi,* or "great sleep," due to septic shock resulting from a blood infection. His legacy is his bold vision of what human beings were capable of—a new world order.

Canadians benefited greatly from this swami choosing Canada as a place to live and inspire, to launch his colourful peace missions from, and to train Canadian teachers for the next generations—you will most likely find one in a neighbourhood near you.

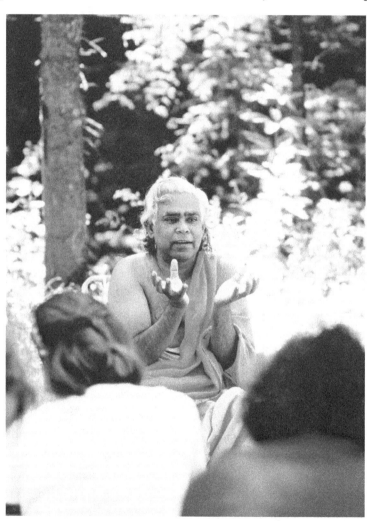

Swami Vishnudevananda, lecturing

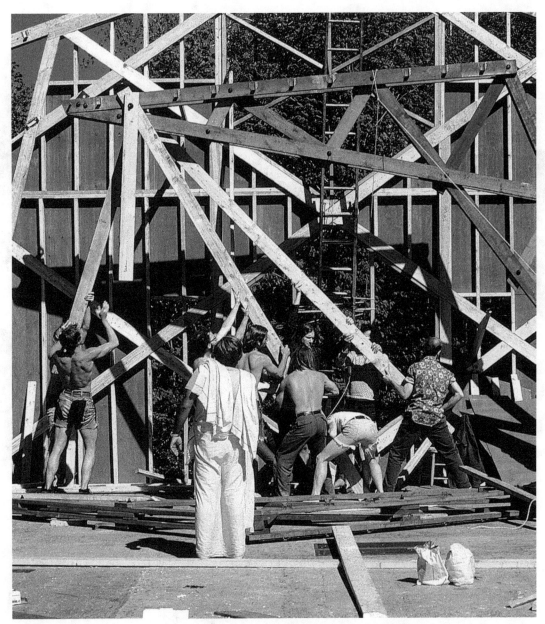

building the ashram at Val Morin, Quebec, 1963

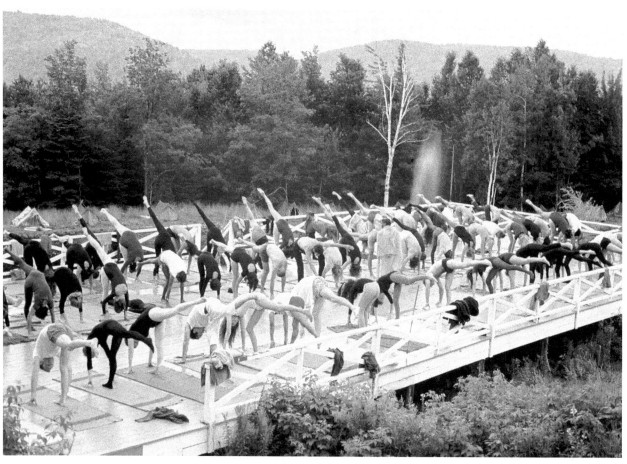

outdoor classes Sivananda Ashram, Val Morin, Quebec

Swami Shraddananda (Claude Passaro)

Born Cavaillon, France, March 1945 –

When Claude was a young man in France, he was curious about the meaning of life. What was our purpose? Why the grand mystery? Why did suffering and joy coexist in the human condition? He was heavily involved in martial arts when, at age eighteen, he was in a serious car accident. Says Claude: "I came out of the car accident miraculously alive, but seriously injured. I started practicing hatha yoga and within a few months, a lot of my form and energy returned. Further, I discovered the intriguing life philosophy attached to yoga. The more I explored it, the more convinced I was on the right path." Claude began studying the Sivananda tradition with well-known Swami Hamsananda, in France. Swami Hamsananda was a pupil of Swami Sivananda in Rishikesh, who took his vows in 1960 and returned to France to teach and serve. It is from this master and lineage that Claude became initiated, receiving the name Swami Shraddananda.

When Swami Shraddananda immigrated to Montreal in 1967, he became the third swami in Canada in the Sivananda lineage, following Swami Radha of Kootenay Bay, British Columbia, and Swami Vishnudevananda of Montreal.

Swami Shraddananda began teaching full time at the Yvon Yva Centre on Palais du Commerce Rue Berri. In the early 1970s, he founded the Lotus Center for the Development of Being, which is still running today. Here, he taught Hatha Yoga classes, but added workshops in Raja Yoga philosophy for personal and spiritual growth. His specific interest was in teaching people how to live more well-rounded lives, engaging life skills that brought good health and joy. A sought-after lecturer and author, Swami Shraddananda has acquired a reputation as a respected and humble leader. In the late 1970s he developed a friendship with Swami Sai Shivananda PhD, another citizen of France who immigrated to Quebec, and Swami Shraddananda became his teacher and mentor. With his support, Swami Shivananda went on to profile French-speaking teachers by founding the noteworthy Francophone Federation of Yoga Teachers.

Says Claude: "My greatest satisfaction is to see within my lifetime how far yoga has spread in the West and to be a part of this extraordinary wave that has genuinely helped improve the lives and health of so many more people. What could be more joyful than this?"

To meet Claude is to meet a quiet-spoken, modest person—in this he embodies the humility of the yoga teachings. He is one of the hidden gems in Canada and one that has admirably represented

French-speaking Canada. In addition to enhancing thousands of lives through his Lotus Centre for the Development of Being, his fifty-year career has trained hundreds of yoga teachers who come from all parts of Canada and France. His skill, experience, and sense of humanity have given countless people inspiration and the tools to live a successful life.

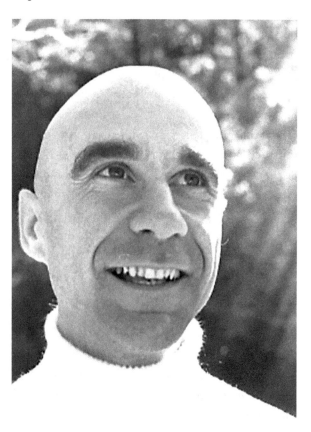

Young Claude Passaro

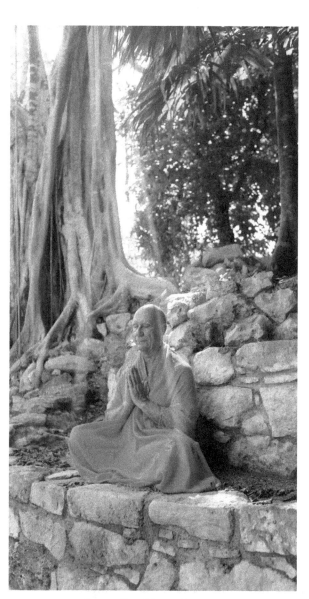

Swami Shraddananda, 2015

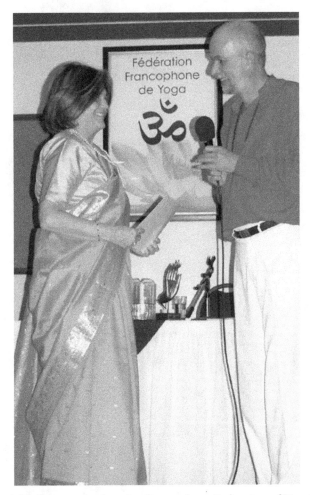

Swami Sai Shivananda, founder, Francophone Federation of Yoga FFY,
awarding Swami Atmajananda

Part 5
Scholars

Who knew that Canada could boast such lofty scholars of yoga? In the 1960s, Canada was a veritable desert as far as yoga philosophy went. Then along came these six scholarly gems to plant the seeds. They were all influenced by yoga in India, most of them at a young age. It shaped their personalities and their destinies. Their love of the ancient scriptures from which yoga philosophy sprang—the *Vedas,* the *Bhagavad Gita*, the *Ramayana*—inspired them. Canadians were fortunate to have these intellectuals among them. They held Westerners' predisposition to practice asana as if it were the sum total of yoga somewhat askance. They were passionate proponents of the Eight Limbs of Yoga in its entirety—a systematic study of the mind. Says Dad Prithipaul: "I felt at times like a lone voice in the wilderness—you cannot do yoga, you can only be yoga. It is a state of mind." Or, as Ravi Ravindra says, "Most people practice yoga today to look sexy, but that is not really yoga." It could, of course, be argued that the Westerner's preoccupation with asana as yoga is, in part, due to the lack of available scholars to teach otherwise. However, despite the belief that the West was embracing yoga superficially, these scholars persevered in their teachings. They saw the *Bhagavad Gita* as a fascinating context from which to understand human suffering, and they saw the *Yoga Sutras of Patanjali* as a timeless recipe for living. Our Canadian scholars have collectively written fifteen internationally acclaimed books. The dial has moved slowly, and today's yoga student is hungry for authentic yoga philosophy and, as ever, there are so few scholars to meet the demand.

Hubert Dhanaraj, PhD

Born South India, 1929; died Edmonton, Alberta, 1993

When the University of Alberta wanted to introduce a PhD program in exercise physiology in 1966, they were looking for someone to fill the position. Upon the recommendation of Professor Mohan Singh, Hubert Dhanaraj came from South India to apply. Said Mohan: "Hubert was immediately accepted upon arrival. He was humble and quiet, a gentleman. He was liked by all."

Hubert was a yoga student in India and didn't waste any time working with Mohan to grow enthusiasm for yoga at U of A. He was encouraged by Mohan to educate Albertans on yoga's benefits. Hubert started by founding the U of A Keep-Fit Yoga Club, where he taught for eighteen years. He went on to publish *Fitness Through Yoga*, becoming the first Canadian to do a research paper and PhD on the physiological effects of yoga.

Hubert worked as a fitness consultant for Alberta Parks and Recreation. His employer was keen to assist Hubert in promoting yoga in the province. Together with Alberta Youth, Culture and Recreation, grants were given and these two organizations financially founded the Yoga Association of Alberta in 1973. The YAA initiative has proved successful, with a large membership and a distinction as Canada's longest-running provincial yoga association.

In 1978, Hubert helped launch the first-ever yoga symposium held at U of A in conjunction with the Commonwealth Games. He also organized the first yoga conference in Alberta, called *Challenge to Change*, in 1981.

Hubert insisted on teaching all aspects of yoga, including yoga as a spiritual discipline. He was one of the first in Alberta to offer meditation classes and a lecture series on the writings of Patanjali—the father of Raja Yoga. Hubert liked to write, "Join the pursuit of excellence in understanding the wise teachings of Patanjali, and in developing comradeship among yoga followers, bound by love and understanding."

Hubert died of cancer in 1993 at age sixty-four.

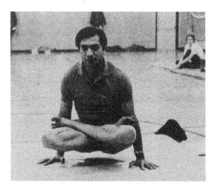

Hubert Dhanaraj, photo: University of Alberta student newspaper

Dad (Dadabhai) Prithipaul, PhD

Born Saint Julien, Mauritius, 1927 –

It would appear that an unseen hand has guided Dad Prithipaul to countries where there was an eager audience for his vast knowledge of Indian philosophies, including Edmonton, Alberta, in 1968.

Dad was the youngest of four boys born to a schoolmaster father in a modest family on the island of Mauritius. His introduction to philosophy was through a few books in his father's library. He met Swami Nihsreyasananda, an accomplished metaphysician of the Ramakrishna Mission. They met for study and discussion on *The Upanishads* for over two years. Although his father died young of an aneurysm, Dad was helped to take further studies at Banaras Hindu University in Varanasi, India when he received one of six fellowships given nationwide. He completed his doctorate at Sorbonne University in Paris.

An opportunity came to lecture at the Center for the Study of World Religions at Harvard University in 1968. While there, he received a phone call offering him an assistant professorship at the University of Alberta, in Edmonton. Prithipaul accepted, making him the first professor in Western Canada to teach the philosophies of India.

Dad gave courses on Hinduism and Buddhism as well as the *Bhagavad Gita* and the *Mandukya Upanishad,* two foundational writings of yoga philosophy. He was also the first professor Canada-wide to teach Western mysticism, a subject that was so specialized that, when he retired, they were unable to fill his spot.

Says Dad on the subject of yoga: "The yoga of Patanjali is the only genuine psychology and is India's gift to humanity. I celebrate Patanjali as the first lover of all living beings, as the provider of the means necessary for the attainment of *moksha,* or of *nirvana,* or of *kaivalya,* that is, of mystic self-fulfillment. Yoga is not an Indian thing—it is a human thing. It is universal, transcending history and geography. It only happens that someone called Patanjali lived in India, hence its origin."

In 1969, Professor Prithipaul joined Professor Mohan Singh at the University of Alberta to found the non-profit Yoga Association of Alberta, and serve as vice-president. Being a scholar amongst an asana-dominant yoga scene at the time, he challenged teachers and students alike to "Keep the yoga in yoga. Every moment is pregnant with the possibility of realization."

Dad went on to publish scholarly works such as *The Labyrinth of Solitude,* a study drawn from the epic work of the *Mahabharata,* and *The Sublime Myth of Rama,* based on the renowned Indian epic the *Ramayana.* He is also known for putting his gift with words into persuasive editorials that challenge social injustices, particularly those done in the name of religion.

Since his retirement, Dad leads informal study groups. His grateful students enjoy his brilliant intellect balanced with his playful humour. Student Carol Fedun describes him as: "A jewel in the crown."

About the unseen guiding hand in his life, Dad comments with his usual dry wit: "There was nothing particular in the entire course of my life. It has been quite banal. I just followed my deep desire to explore the mysteries of philosophical thought. I did this despite all the advices to the contrary. I was a lone traveler, but it was all a blessing."

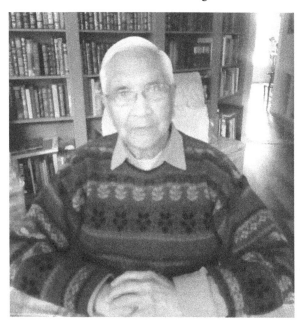

Dad Prithipaul, Edmonton, Alberta, 2017

Ravi Ravindra, PhD

Born Sunam, India, 1938 –

Ravi taught his first yoga class when a professor at Dalhousie University in Halifax, Nova Scotia, in 1966. Later, he was to lament this effort as ineffective. "People were practicing yoga as a body movement, to be more sexy, and not to seek spiritual advancement," he recalls. It confirmed for him the kind of teacher he wanted to be.

Ravi received his PhD in physics from the University of Toronto and is a professor emeritus of comparative religion and philosophy from Dalhousie University. Although an accomplished academic with several degrees, Ravi defines himself more as a relentless seeker of truth through mysticism and spirituality. It is from this role as a seeker that he feels he has made the most significant contribution to his fellow man. His role of urging others to take on spiritual inquiry began due to two early childhood experiences.

The first is when, as a young boy in India, he would watch his father joyfully delve into holy books and poetry for hours. He remembers one day vividly as his father quoted a passage from the *Bhagavad Gita* that said, "At the end of many births, a wise person comes to me realizing that all there is is Krishna. Such a person

is a great soul and very rare." He then turned to Ravi and said, "You know, Ravi, I know what these words say, but I don't know what they really mean. I hope you will find a teacher or teaching that will assist you to understand its real meaning."

That moment, Ravi's lifelong quest to find Krishna was sparked.

The second was when Ravi was nine years old and his country was in the Indo-Pakistani War and being divided into Pakistan and India. He witnessed mayhem and mass murder in the streets below his home.

After the events and in one of those rare moments that move inner mountains, Ravi witnessed his father, a Hindu, reunite with an old neighbour, a Muslim. He describes what took place: "It was to be an unforgettable experience for me. Before any words were spoken, my father and his old neighbour embraced each other for fifteen minutes. They were crying loudly and unable to utter a single word. It broke my heart."

These experiences were traumatic for Ravi. They also struck him as confusing—how could religion espouse the highest in man, the Krishna, and yet also evoke the cruelest of actions?

If this suffering was wrought from religion, where was the divine mystery to all life to be found? What was truth?

Thus, simultaneous with his academic career as a professor, Ravi sought out teachers who would help him in his search. He had a personal relationship with philosopher Jiddu Krishnamurti, who taught him that no one had a monopoly on truth. He had a close relationship with TKV Desikachar of India, who helped him with yoga asana practice. He delved into the *Yoga Sutras of Patanjali*, which state that attachment to beliefs, even if it is religion, is still an attachment and thus causes suffering. Further influences came with mystic George Gurdjieff, studies in Zen, and the great Hindu and Christian mystics. All of these convinced Ravi that nothing replaced direct experience obtained from open inquiry, and that this direct experience superseded any doctrine.

As Ravi merged these teachings with his academic and personal life, he wrote about his understandings in several books: *A Guide to the Bhagavad Gita, The Yoga of Christ,* and *The Wisdom of the Yoga Sutras of Patanjali.* He has written over 100 articles and publications on spirituality.

Ravi is quick to recognize in others the same hunger for spiritual understanding he has had all his life. Thus, he continues to give of his time generously through international speaking engagements and webinars.

Says Ravi from his home in Nova Scotia: "Here and there I encounter serious searchers and I am happy to share with them what I understand the great teachers have said in well-known texts. If I can actually practice one instruction of the Buddha or the Christ or Krishna, that is more important to me than what a hundred philosophers or theologians have to say. I am more a searcher than a scholar, but I have nothing against scholars or scholarship."

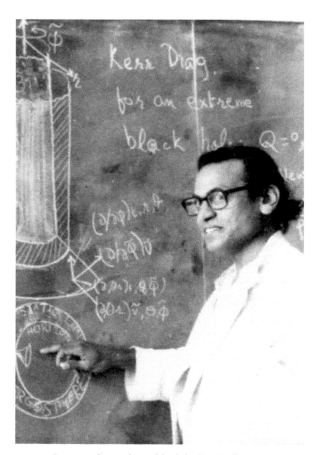

Ravi teaching about black holes, Dalhousie University, 1969

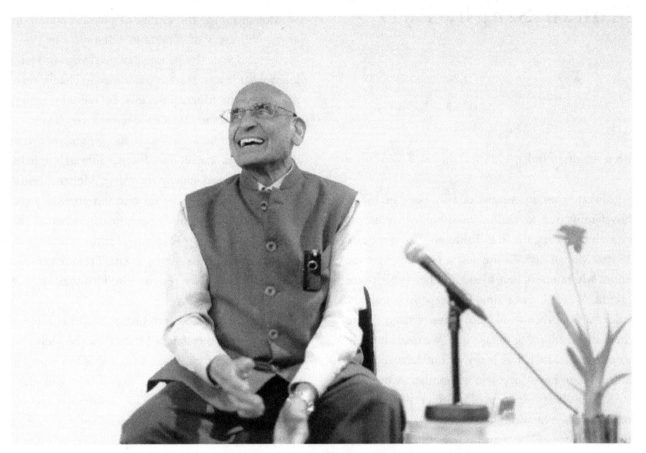

Ravi Ravindra 2016, sage and scholar

Mohan Singh, PhD

Born Amritsar, India, 1931 –

Mohan grew up surrounded by yoga in India. His family was to endure hardship when it lost everything during the Indo-Pakistani War in the late 1940s. Mohan says, "I was just a boy and we were Sikhs. My mother's best friend and her family were Hindu. When it came time to escape in a military truck, my mother would not leave, stating, 'Take them if you are going to take me.' We made it safely to our destination, but many of our relatives were killed. I have never forgotten my mother's words."

Mohan later experienced another life-defining moment when he was filling in a college application that asked for his permanent address. "It really hit me in that moment—I had no permanent address and we had lost everything. It was a devastating feeling I can still feel today." Despite the hardship, Mohan completed a master's degree and stayed to teach in India. He then earned a US-sponsored Fulbright Scholarship to do a PhD in physiology in Springfield, Massachusetts. While there, he taught yoga at the local YMCA. It was here his interest in yoga as a life practice grew.

Mohan joined the faculty of physical education at the University of Alberta in Edmonton in 1966. He noticed very few people practiced yoga or really knew what it was. He was passionate to change that. As part of the fitness programs, he started teaching free yoga classes to drum up interest, later charging a nominal fee of fifty cents per class. These classes were the first yoga classes in Alberta, although Friedel Khattab followed shortly thereafter. Mohan pressed for the university to set up credit courses in yoga, which they did, becoming the first in Alberta. The classes were called" Yoga for Health and Fitness" and "Yoga for Stress Management." The first course filled with over sixty people. These courses are still running today.

Mohan mentored promising student Hubert Dhanaraj to gather scientific data on the merits of yoga and present it to the public. He felt that people were more likely to take up yoga if they had more information on its benefits. This resulted in Hubert completing a PhD on the physical benefits of yoga in 1973. The dissertation was published and is still available at the U of A library.

Both Mohan and Hubert went on to found the non-profit Yoga Association of Alberta in 1976, an organization that shows impressive longevity. They started the organization to obtain government grants for yoga programs. Mohan became its first president and served on the board of the YAA until his retirement in 1996.

In the late 1980s, Mohan was part of a group of professors tasked with developing a physical fitness program for the Department of National Defense for its soldiers. A five-year government grant was given to set performance standards. Breathing and meditation were introduced with significant performance improvement noted from the meditation and included as part of the published study.

As Mohan reflects on his half century in Edmonton, he says, "Canada gave me a home again—it replaced what I had lost. It warms my heart. I am grateful for its beauty and I am even more grateful to have made a contribution to yoga education in Alberta."

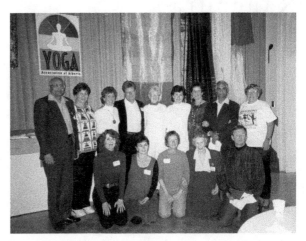

YAA – AGM, 1996; back row: Mohan Singh, Susan Blackner, Shirley Johannesen, Chris Robinson, Hilda Pezarro, Val Petrich, Grace Little, Dad Prithipaul, Friedel Khattab,
Front row: Bonnie Dunbar, Sarah Wilson, Mary Leblanc Kay Sherman, David McAmmond

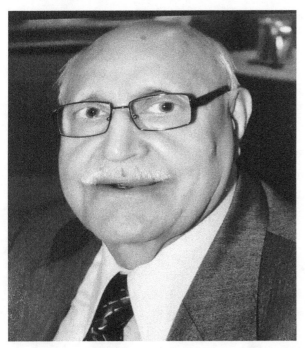

Mohan Singh, Edmonton, Alberta, 2018

Ranendra Sinha, PhD

Born Purbadhala, India (now Bangladesh), 1930;
died Winnipeg, Manitoba, 2013

Ranen was nineteen and a pre-med student in Calcutta, India, in 1946 during the Indian partition riots. He was traumatized by the violence and death he witnessed in the streets and this influenced his life-long search for spiritual meaning through the teachings of yoga.

He devoured ancient yoga philosophical texts and meditated for long hours, even while completing a master's degree in zoology and anatomy at the University of Calcutta. Leaving India, he completed a PhD in entomology in Kansas before immigrating to Winnipeg, Canada, in 1978.

Ranen excelled in his field as a world expert on the protective storage of grain from microflora and pests. He spoke at conferences worldwide and spent a year in Japan as a consultant. However, at heart he was a devoted yogi and scholar of yoga philosophy. The karma yoga thoughts instilled in him by his father and witnessing of man's inhumanity to man in wartime India created a deep yearning for spiritual knowledge. He found it through the writings of Shankarya and Vedanta yoga philosophy and his greatest passion was to share it. He had no formal yoga teacher or lineage and was largely self-taught. He was nevertheless passionate and articulate and his classes were so popular they typically ran full with a waitlist. He eventually wrote a book called *Yoga: Two Concepts and Four Choices,* which was published by the University of Manitoba.

Ranen was dismayed that there was so much emphasis on yoga as postures. He took it as a personal mission to enrich people's understanding of yoga by teaching the broad philosophy of the Eight Limbs of Yoga. During his two-hour classes, he would lecture on the philosophy of yoga first and devote the second hour to asana, pranayama, and meditation.

Ranen taught at community centres, schools, and the continuing education department of the University of Manitoba. He founded the Yoga Society of Manitoba in the early 1980s as a way to encourage fellowship in yoga. When Ranen passed away, he left behind many grateful, lifelong students who remember him as a man who lived a disciplined life and who applied his faith in yoga philosophy to live each day consciously. People would remark that even his strolls in the evening were important to him to make meaningful connections to people. In him, they found a friend who was always keen to not waste a minute but to communicate his deepest thoughts and feelings and to let people know he prayed for them every day.

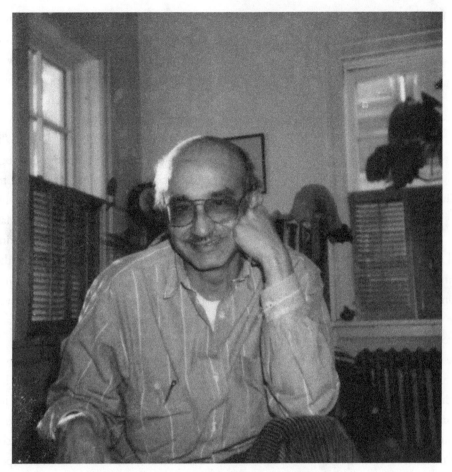

Ranen Sinha, 1988 Winnipeg, Manitoba

Norman Sjoman, PhD

Born Mission City, British Columbia, 1944 –

One of the world's foremost Sanskrit scholars is Canadian and he resides in Calgary, Alberta. His impressive contributions to scholarly material on yoga have been noted in the *Encyclopedia of Indian Philosophy, Vol. 13*. Norman studied at the University of British Columbia, Vancouver before heading to Stockholm University. While there, he picked up a book by Bishnu Charan Ghosh and taught himself headstands. He had begun studying Sanskrit and met an older Indian named Chandrakant Desai who introduced him to the oral aspect of Sanskrit and started him memorizing large amounts of material in Sanskrit.

Chandrakant helped Norman register at Pune University in India to further his studies. He stayed in Pune from 1970 to 1976, obtaining a PhD in Sanskrit from the Centre of Advanced Studies. During those seven years, Norman studied yoga daily with BKS Iyengar. This was years before Westerners sought out Mr. Iyengar and he had not yet become famous. Norman gained a depth of understanding about asana and pranayama from him that lasted a lifetime and gave him rare preparation as a teacher.

Norman credits Mr. Iyengar with launching a modern tradition of yoga defined by what he called "the balance and precision he brought to his work." Norman further credits Mr. Iyengar's book, *Light on Yoga*, first published in 1965, with "bringing a new thoroughness and objectivity to yoga, making it a reference book for all of asana done today."

After moving to Mysore, Norman obtained a pandit degree from the Mysore Maharaja's Mahapathasala. He stayed to do research in Mysore, taking an interest in unpublished manuscripts. He found the *Sritattvanidhi*, a text with 122 asanas from the nineteenth century that had no clear lineage or tradition; he determined a clear influence of British gymnastics and other exercise systems, including the use of ropes. This curriculum and gymnasium with ropes were passed on to Tirumalai Krishnamacharya in the 1920s when he arrived as yoga teacher to the Mysore palace. Sri Krishnamacharya was to gain fame as the teacher to Mr. Iyengar as well as Pattabhi Jois and Krishnamacharya's son TKV Desikachar. These three teachers spearheaded yoga's explosion in the West.

Norman's research and publication, *The Yoga Tradition of the Mysore Palace,* was published in 1996, upsetting some yoga practitioners who felt they had the authentic handle on yoga from the gurus. However, it awakened serious academic scholarship on yoga and initiated a whole flock of modern studies on the origin of asanas. Sjoman's 2013 book, *Yogasutracintamani*, has taken that study to a whole new level by considering traditional Sanskrit scholarship in application to actual practice.

He has also made an impressive contribution to scholarly material on yoga noted in the 2011 publication, *Encyclopedia of Indian Philosophies Vol. XIII.*

Although Norman returned to the West at times to teach at various universities such as the University of California, Berkeley, the University of British Columbia, the University of Calgary, and so on, he always kept a home in south Mysore, India.

In addition to Sanskrit studies, Norman completed an art degree at Southern Alberta Institute of Art in Calgary in 1990. He published books on South Indian music, artists in Mysore, and artists at large, and has written numerous catalogues for artists in India and Sri Lanka. He brings yoga into his own sculpture, painting, and textile art and some of his personal art collection has been exhibited publicly.

About the philosophy of yoga and his lifetime of scholarly works, Norman says: "Yoga is really a spiritual discipline for accessing consciousness efficiently. The Sutras of Patanjali explain the means of accomplishment. Some people are born with this ability, others get it through drugs, some people get it through chanting, others the death process, and so on. However, the Sutras delineate a pathway. It is through yoga you can learn to purify your karma, the residue we leave to the next generation through our actions."

Norman resides in Calgary where he still teaches classes in advanced asana. When not hiking or on his motorcycle, he is cooking Indian dishes for his many visitors. He continues to travel and accept speaking and teaching engagements from a worldwide network of fellow travelers on the path.

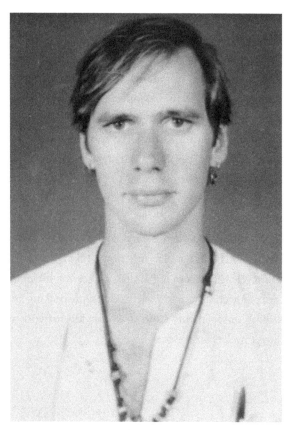

Norman Sjoman, Sanskrit scholar, Pune, India, 1967

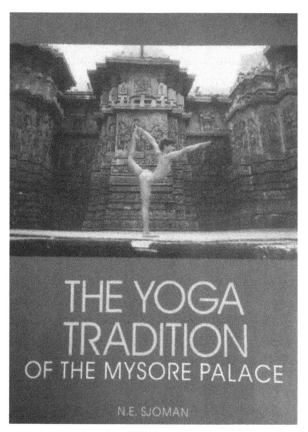

THE YOGA
TRADITION
OF THE MYSORE PALACE

N.E. SJOMAN

Norman Sjoman, scholarly work

Part 6
Visionaries

These pioneer yogis stand out as visionaries because of experiences with the paranormal. These experiences shaped their lives as luminaries, or ones who shine light on the path for others. Their experiences are varied—a near-death experience, prophetic dreams, nudges from guardian angels, and information "channeled" to them to write a book. Some of them shared with me that, at times, they had a sense of being instruments of a grander design. They, in turn, trusted the message and responded to it as a personal calling. In rising to the occasion, they showed a lot of courage. Ultimately, it resulted in worthwhile work for their fellow beings. For some of these teachers, yoga as a study of mysticism, spectra of consciousness, and reincarnation provided a context from which to understand their visionary experiences. When interviewing these people, I noted their willingness to pay attention to synchronicity in their lives, seeing events not as random but intricately connected for a purpose. As they practiced this attention to detail with others in their daily lives, they noticed they felt led to being part of a bigger picture. Like all of the other pioneers in this book, they stayed curious to the mystical aspects of yoga and sourced out books, teachers, and each other to help understand the subtleties that presented through their practice. These are our visionaries.

Patricia Dewar

Born Edmonton, Alberta, 1938 –

In 1971, Patricia was a young, vibrant thirty-three-year-old teaching dance at Laurentian University in Sudbury, Ontario, when her life took a drastic turn. She ended up in the intensive care ward with extensive internal injuries after being seriously injured in a car accident. She almost died.

By her own account, she had a near-death experience (NDE) that shaped her life profoundly. Says Patricia: "I sensed a universal law, that the body is not only defined by gravity, but more importantly, the body is electric. Love and light surrounded me."

Her route to recovery was long and arduous. The physio sessions felt mechanical and left her feeling dissatisfied. Her subsequent recovery and spiritual search led to her to become the first therapeutic yoga teacher of her kind in Saskatchewan.

She started with studies "to understand the body as a transformational tool," in such diverse body disciplines as modern dance, choreography, dance ethnography, Feldenkrais, the Alexander Technique, and somatic studies. During these years Patricia earned a bachelor of physical education, a bachelor of arts, a master's of science with a dance major, and a PhD from the University of Alberta

In Patricia's words, "I likened my life to a moth circling around the flame. I was seeking a rediscovery of that early experience of inner light."

She stumbled on a yoga class on campus. The view of body as the temple of spirit appealed to her, as did the practice of poses in stillness with a meditative mind. The practice of *savasana*, (deep relaxation pose) brought a profound recall of her NDE. She knew now she was in familiar territory and she felt safe to explore it.

When she moved to Saskatoon and taught the history of dance at the University of Saskatchewan, she began teaching yoga classes to the public on the side. She had recently stumbled upon the Iyengar style of yoga and the depth and accuracy appealed to her. She started attending Jo-Ann Sutherland's yoga studio in Saskatoon, and began teaching there. She also obtained an advanced teaching certificate from Donald Moyer at the Yoga Room in Berkeley, California. Moving into full-time teaching, Patricia opened the Yoga Central Studio in Saskatoon in 2000, thus taking Saskatchewan forward in the availability of therapeutic yoga and meditation. She gained a reputation as a compassionate teacher and trainer who possessed an intuitive gift to help people in recovery. Yoga Central closed in 2011.

"Life for me is no longer about finding meaning. Now I realize life is a wondrous, magical gift of being. Intuitively, even before my accident, I sensed how fragile and precious life could be. But the spiritual experience entails the body-felt sense of knowing that I am part of this Divine Light. The gift of being born human is the gift of conscious choice. And so, like the moth around the flame, I engaged in my life's journey to feel the touch of the Spirit on the Body."

A diagnosis of leukemia has not dimmed Patricia's light. She radiates an aura of serenity that makes you want to be in her presence. *Yoga Journal* recently chose her for a pilot study on energy medicine yoga in California.

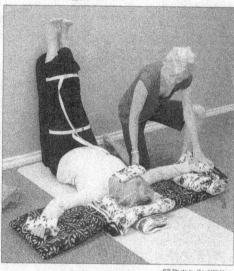

...atoon, Saskatchewan   TheStarPhoenix.com   **LOCAL A7**

s healing continue

to get more
r movement,"

...cer, she has
...portunities
...port groups,
...asses, her
. most recently,
...C Run for the
...port came from
...p Centre at the

...ed to get
...it. I always
...cancer, but
...me," she said.
...use I had to."
...divorce dur-
...y lives in a
...rge abstract
...walls. She's
...again.
...u get better,"
...hoice."
...rogram is
...adian Breast
...nce and the
...Centre at the
...ticipants. The
...an. 6. For more
...earcher Susan
...ertson@
...076.
...est.com

—SP Photo by Gord Waldner
Instructor Patricia Dewar (right) helps a student achieve a yoga position

Patricia Dewar; photo: *Saskatoon Star Phoenix*

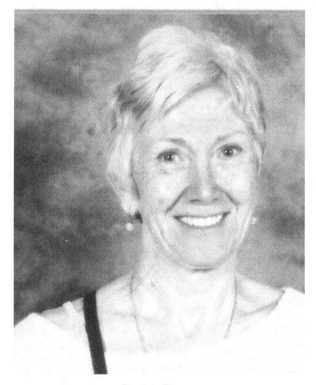

Patricia Dewar

David Edney

Born Kingston, Ontario, 1942 –

At the youthful age of seventy-one, David Edney was the first to bring yoga to Saskatchewan prisons.

A retired professor of language at the University of Saskatchewan, Saskatoon, David was listening to a radio interview in 2011 that criticized inmates for being "gifted" with things such as exercise classes. A firm believer in rehabilitation, David was dismayed. He then reflected—maybe there was something he could to add to their lives. In that moment, he had a sudden burst of clarity. He attributes it to his guardian angel, whom he says nudges him at important times in his life. He knew it was yoga he wanted to share.

David had started off with Kareen Zebroff's books over thirty years earlier and had a committed home practice. But now he knew he had to become an instructor. So while living in Kingston, Ontario, to be with his ailing mother, David signed up for a yoga teacher training program. He was the only male in the class. Coincidentally, his father had worked in administration at the Collins Bay Penitentiary near Kingston, and David clearly remembered a tour his father gave him when he was ten years old.

In his teacher training course, David pivoted. "I was torn between excitement about all this wonderful stuff I was learning, and embarrassment about this idea of me, a frail, old academic thinking of teaching inmates in a jail." He got cold feet and temporarily changed his focus to yoga with seniors.

Nonetheless, when David returned to Saskatoon with his teacher certificate in hand, he enrolled in an Indigenous studies course and was inspired by the guest lecturer who spoke specifically on Indigenous peoples in jail. It captured his interest sufficiently to revive his old plan, and he contacted the Saskatoon Correctional Centre.

Thus, David is credited with being the first to offer yoga classes in a penal setting in Saskatchewan.

Nothing is more powerful than an idea whose time had come—David went further with a vision of helping to train Indigenous yoga teachers in Saskatchewan to take yoga to their communities and to their population in jail. David saw the strong connection between yoga and traditional Indigenous world views.

"The holistic view of the person—physical, mental, emotional, spiritual—it's the medicine wheel, and that corresponds very much to the yoga view of all of these aspects forming an organic whole, making up the person and their relationship to the community and the world," he explains.

In 2016, David partnered with the Saskatoon Tribal Council to offer a scholarship program. When applicants came forward, both Indigenous and non-Indigenous, David then created the Saskatchewan Indigenous Yoga Association. Says David: "In little over a year, the accomplishments of SIYA have been impressive—six scholarships awarded, three new teachers taking yoga to Indigenous communities, four support grants awarded, a teacher-training workshop given, and an organization set up with an Indigenous-dominated executive and an Indigenous chair. The potential for the future is limitless. All my own efforts to bring this about led to nothing. Only when I found the right contact so that action could go forward under indigenous leadership were there any results."

David had such conviction over the value of the project that he financed it. "I've been blessed with a well-paying job and an inheritance from my parents and I have far more than I would ever need myself. It's not any virtue on my part to accumulate possessions. That's of no interest to me," he says. "I have no dependents. I'm free to do this stuff, which is extremely gratifying. I have planted the seed money and got something started so it can become independent. It was all part of listening to my guardian angel."

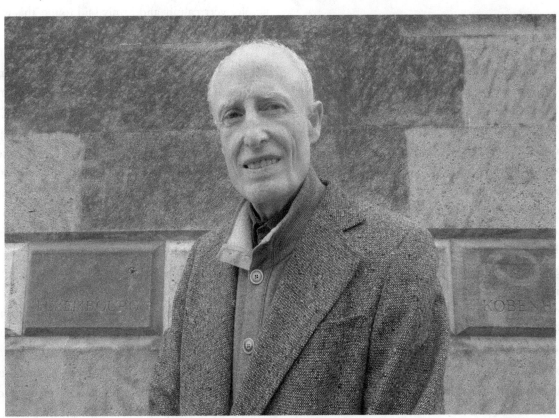

David Edney, Saskatoon, Saskatchewan, founder of SIYA

Guru Raj Kaur Khalsa

Born Brooklyn, New York, 1951 –

Margaret Mary Polemis is one of the longest-serving women in the 3HO tradition (Healthy, Happy, Holy). She was set to go on a European bike tour with her brother in the fall of 1971 when fate intervened. She was invited to check out a 3HO Kundalini yoga class and she liked it so much she committed to a forty-day practice of *sat kriya*. Says Margaret: "That was it! This experience awakened my destiny. I was 'in' and I was committed. I never did the bike trip and I never looked back."

Margaret then met Yogi Bhajan, the founder of 3HO, while attending a seven-day winter solstice gathering in Florida. A Sikh from India, Yogi Bhajan experienced an early spiritual awakening that inspired him to start teaching in the West. She says of their meeting: "When I arrived at his first class, I suddenly saw on the stage an image of a man with a long beard and soulful eyes, rather than Yogi Bhajan. When my vision cleared, I saw it actually was Yogi Bhajan. I discovered later that the first face I saw was that of Guru Ram Dass, the fourth Sikh Guru who

lived 400 years ago, who Yogi Bhajan always said he was in service to. That experience taught me humility and what it means to trust a lineage and serve a legacy."

Margaret devoted herself to the lineage and was given the name Guru Raj Kaur Khalsa, which means "princess who establishes the rule of wisdom." Guru Raj's calling was later confirmed during a meditation. She recalls: "It was as if all the veils of my ego parted. It's hard to put into words, but what I call my soul's voice very calmly and firmly said to me 'this will do,' meaning 'this is a worthy path to follow.' That voice has stayed with me my whole life and I have allowed it to lead me. I teach my students to trust hearing the voice of their soul over their ego, and then muster the courage to follow it."

In 1972, Guru Raj Kaur married a young man named Guru Raj Singh (Michael North), who was also part of the new 3HO community in Toronto. With others, they founded the first ashram at 333 Palmerston Boulevard. When they chanced to be in Vancouver that year, they fell in love with it. Leaving the Toronto ashram in the hands of Guru Tej Singh and Guru Tej Kaur, they moved to Vancouver to establish a 3HO community. They soon rented space in Kitsilano, calling it the New Age Community Centre, and launched a newspaper that became a glossy magazine called *New Directions*.

Since 1986, Guru Raj Kaur and her current husband, Hari Singh, another early member of the Toronto ashram, have devoted their lives to creating a successful studio and harmonious community in

Vancouver through Yoga West in Kitsilano, where they remain teaching today.

Guru Raj Kaur wrote and delivers an internationally recognized teacher training curriculum, and, along with her senior teachers, graduates over forty teachers annually.

In the 1990s, Guru Raj Kaur founded the Khalsa Ladies Summer Camp, a gathering of women for spiritual practice and fellowship that continues to this day. Her two daughters attended each year, one starting at age three! They grew up to become accomplished yoga teachers in their own right.

Still going strong after forty-five years of service, Guru Raj Kaur has earned a reputation as a loving and wise teacher. Part of her timeless appeal has been her acts of selflessness, as well as her compassion for a troubled world. "When you teach from your pure essence, your ego gets weeded out. Then there is nothing loud anymore—no trumpets, just a soft gratitude. When your subconscious is clear, acts of grace can come in. Believe it and trust it. Then go do your life with this gift. It doesn't really matter what tradition you choose. It can be the 'this will do' defining moment like I had. It only matters that you have a spiritual practice and shift your own consciousness in order to change the world and bring peace."

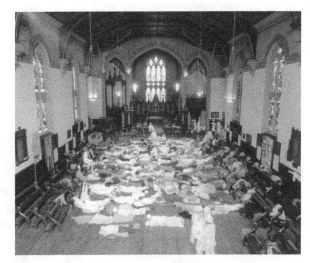

3HO meditation at Church of Holy Trinity, Toronto, 1970s

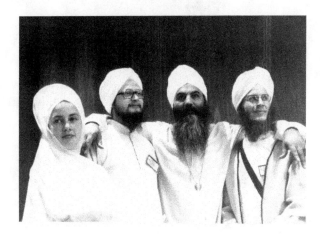

Guru Raj Kaur Khalsa, Michael North, Yogi Bhajan and Ted Steiner

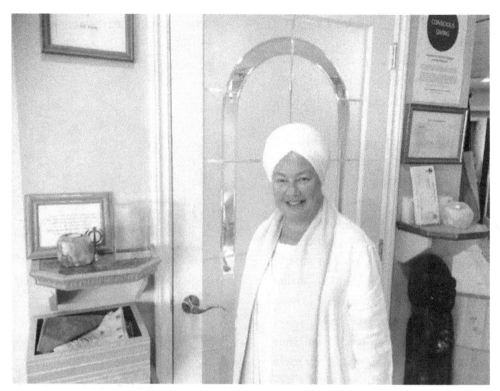

Guru Raj Kaur Khalsa, Yoga West, Vancouver,
British Columbia, 2017

Divya Prabha

Born Halifax, Nova Scotia, 1943 –

Divya Prabha opened the first yoga centre in the Maritimes in 1977 and gave her first teacher training program in 1995. She is Canada's first award-winning author and expert on the science of chanting.

Perhaps more importantly, Divya has become a beacon for women on the spiritual path, born out of her extraordinary visionary experiences and her wisdom gained from many years with Indian gurus.

As a child, Divya, née Sally Thompson, always felt she had a destiny to help others. At age twenty-eight, she underwent a three-day spontaneous *kundalini* awakening that resulted in a profound spiritual transformation. It was only later, through finding a book by Gopi Krishna about kundalini awakenings, that she understood what had happened to her. She had received warning of the event the night before it happened through a person she had barely met with a strong psychic gift who was guided to deliver to her a number of messages from the beyond that forewarned of the coming event. He reassured her that she would be taken care of throughout by her maternal grandmother. She was also told that she would have two dreams explaining what was happening to her. One dream involved a huge snake, which opened its mouth wide and hissed a powerful stream of energy directly at her, and the other dream involved the often unnoticed lineage of women—the fact that a woman comes out of a woman who comes out of a woman back to the beginning. A few hours later, the spontaneous orgasms began, wave after wave, which became terrifyingly painful. Just as she feared the worst, a voice spoke to her, saying, "The world is in a very bad way and energy is being given to certain people so that it will survive." That was enough for Divya to hear to allow her to welcome the energy. When the crucial point came where she felt she would die if it didn't stop, she called out for mercy and immediately the stabbing waves of energy subsided. It resulted in realizations of the meaning of existence and the singular importance of the power of love, which filled her with excruciating bliss.

After the event, Divya experienced such a heightened level of energy that it caused a burning sensation, which was only relieved by intense physical activity. Not a very physically active person by nature, she realized she needed to take up a practice of some kind and settled on something she really knew nothing about—yoga asana. Luckily, she found one of the few teachers in the area and began a fervent practice, which led her eventually to take the basic and advanced teacher training at the Kripalu Centre which at the time, was in Pennsylvania with Yogi Amrit Desai presiding. During the advanced training, Yogi Amrit Desai's guru came from India and, when Divya saw him, she recognized him as her spiritual guide. She was fortunate to be one of the very few accepted by Swami Kripalvananda as a disciple, and he initiated her as Divya Prabha (which in Sanskrit means a swift explosion of divine light). This inspired her to start the first yoga centre in Halifax, in 1977, called the Kripalu Yoga Society. It employed six yoga teachers and offered weekly *satsangs* and workshops.

Divya remained devoted to Kripaluji until he died in 1982. Says Divya, "When he took *mahasamadhi*—when a realized soul consciously leaves the body—in India, he gave me three great blessings the night he departed. The next day, I received the call that he was gone, but I knew already."

Divya's second guru was Swami Haridhos Giri of Chennai, India, a major advocate of *kirtan* chanting as a spiritual pathway. His life's work was to revive the practice in India and abroad and his influence on Divya musically was substantial. For several years, she travelled with him extensively. She has since published several popular CDs on Sanskrit chanting.

Divya's third guru was Sri Sri Ravi Shankar, whom she met on his first trip to Canada in 1986. Becoming a loyal devotee, Divya threw all her talents into helping establish his Art of Living Foundation in Canada, the US, India, and abroad. She led the first Art of Living International Teacher Training Program in Bangalore, India, which included the science of chanting as an integral part of the curriculum. After eighteen years of service, she withdrew from Art of Living and lives quietly by the ocean, composing Sanskrit chants and offering rare satsangs at her much-loved Shining Bay Retreat. A collection of her chants is currently in the works, many of which have already been embraced worldwide.

To meet Divya is to have an experience of Mother Earth pulling you into her warmth. This comes through in her book, *Kirtan—the Art and Ecstasy of Chanting,* published in 2016 and a gold award winner in the Nautilus Book Awards. In it, she shares a lifetime of direct experience and brings a rare esoteric subject to life. Her book covers wise topics important to yoga teachers: the meaning of deities, the path of Bhakti devotion, the true meaning of OM, and the power of vibration on our cellular being.

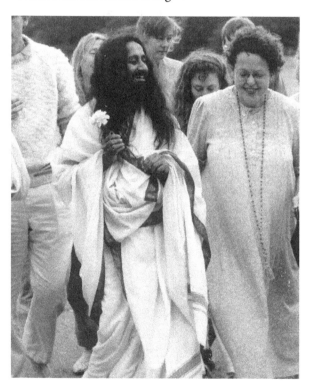

Divya Prabha with Ravi Shankar

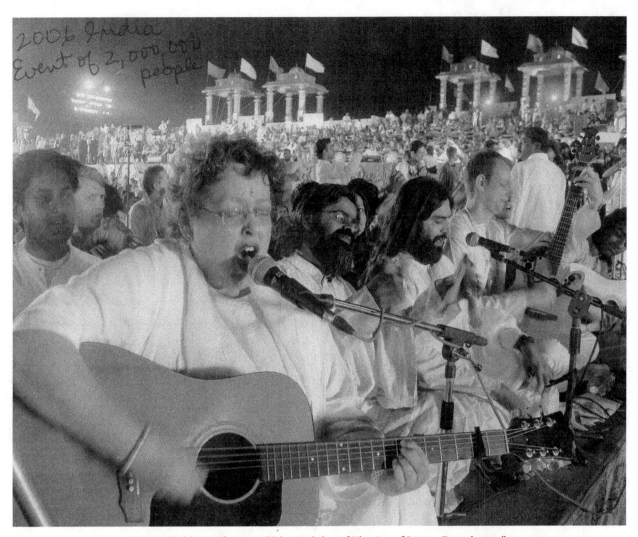

Divya Prabha performing "Silver Jubilee of The Art of Living Foundation,"
two million people attending in Bangalore, India

Marilyn Rossner

Born Montreal, Quebec, date unknown –

When asked about her birthdate, Marilyn says, "I am as young as a blade of grass and as old as eternity."

Marilyn was one of the earliest teachers of the Sivananda method of yoga in Canada. She dedicated her life to yoga and healing others following messages she received as a child. Marilyn was not an average child—she was born with unique visionary gifts.

She was born in Montreal to a family touched by the Holocaust and who followed a strict Kabalarian tradition. Her psychic gifts alarmed her parents, who took her to their rabbi. Luckily, the rabbi recognized her gifts and implored her family to be patient. He described her gifts as "saintly guidance."

Among the many clairvoyant experiences she had as a child was a recurring vision of a bald-headed man who danced with children from around the world. He gave her words to sing in a language she did not know and he gave her a clear message—that her path was to be with children to help ease their suffering.

All of this came to be true.

The message was to return to Marilyn over and over again in her childhood. But it was years later, in 1962, when she walked into the Sivananda Vedanta Centre in Montreal, that it all made sense.

The director of the centre was Swami Vishnudevananda. Behind him on the wall she saw a picture of a bald-headed man that she instantly recognized as the man in her vision. This was Swami Sivananda Sarasvati of the Divine Light Mission. Still alive in Rishikesh, India, Swami Sivananda was a physician, guru, and beloved master of many, often called the "Assisi of India." He had sent his disciple, Swami Vishnudevananda, to the West to spread the teachings of yoga and meditation.

For Marilyn, this was a profound moment, and an affirmation of her life path. She began a long and enduring relationship with Swami Vishnudevananda that lasted until his death in 1993.

When Swami Vishnudevananda set up the Sivananda children and youth camps in Val Morin, Quebec, he chose Marilyn as the ideal candidate to be in charge. As a faculty member and behavioural therapist at Vanier College in Montreal for thirty-five years, her academic understanding combined with her gift as an intuitive healer were well respected. Swami Vishnudevananda referred to Marilyn as a *mahasiddha*, a yogini with exceptional powers. The children's camps were crowded mat-to-mat every summer. Marilyn called on other Canadian yoga teachers as helpers and some returned faithfully each year to work with children and teens, many of whom had special needs. She believed that that some of those with psychiatric issues were actually in spiritual crisis and she was able to guide them. Some of these experiences were included in her thesis and later published in her book *Yoga, Psychotherapy and Children.*

Marilyn accompanied Swami Vishnudevananda on many of the peace missions to trouble spots throughout the world that earned him a reputation as a peacemaker. Says Marilyn:

"Every country we went to there were lineups to see him. Jews, nuns, everyone wanted knowledge from him."

Their famous fire walking in India in the 1980s has been much-recorded; their mission was to prove that mind could triumph over matter, that peace could triumph over hostility. She helped establish many successful interfaith conferences worldwide on topics of spiritual dialogue and yoga and psychic development.

Marilyn spent two years in Russia giving intensive training to a group of psychiatrists on treatment for exceptional children and youth. She taught them how to use traditional yoga, meditation, pranayama, and intuition in their healing. She worked at Mother Teresa's house in Calcutta, and had a special audience with Pope John Paul, who affirmed her selfless work.

In a series of synchronistic events that were to define her life, Marilyn met and married Dr. John Rossner. Soulmates in the true sense of the word, they were married for forty years, until his death in 2014. Rossner was a PhD and ordained Anglican priest who taught religion at Concordia University for forty years. Shaped by his own intuitive experiences, he shared Marilyn's belief that heaven and earth were accessible to all if they simply attuned themselves to the paranormal. Together, they were known as the "introspective and intellectual Anglican priest and a young charismatic Jewish visionary." As part of a prominent worldwide order of notable spiritualists, scientists, and philosophers, they established the Spiritual Science Fellowship. Throughout their entire lives, they remained Sivananda teachers and devotees.

Marilyn works tirelessly to bring people together for what she sees as nothing short of a world paradigm shift. She hosts the successful Spiritual Science Fellowship conferences in Montreal every year, as she has for the last forty-three years, encouraging professionals to meet "for the harmonious integration of science and spirituality." Her talks, books, seminars, and mentorship carry the predominant theme of yoga as a spiritual science. She has been a light giving hope, faith, and courage to thousands of souls in many nations, races, religions, and cultures.

One Montreal reporter said of Marilyn, "You cannot not like her! She is a veritable 'miniature neon-hipster,' this little whirling dervish of a medium."

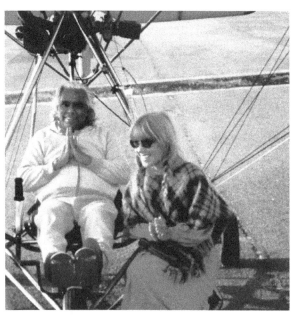

Swami Vishnudevananda with Marilyn Rossner,
preparing for flying mission

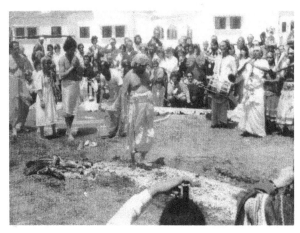

Marilyn and John Rossner firewalking with Swamiji,
India, 1984

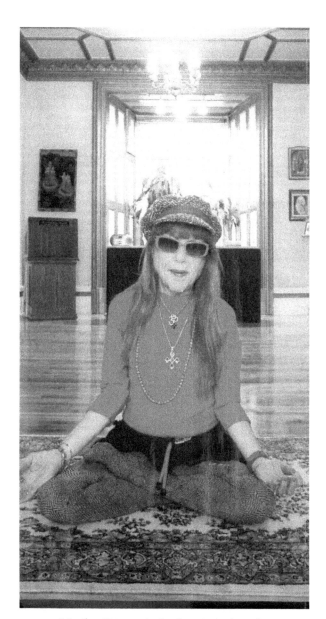

Marilyn Rossner in La Semaine; photo by
Georges Dutil

Kareen Zebroff

Born Heidelberg, Germany, 1941–

Kareen is considered the quintessential First Lady of Yoga in Canada. Her swami once told her that her name means "please do it" in Sanskrit.

Kareen's CTV series, from 1970 to 1986, reached a broad audience across Canada and the northern US, getting thousands of people "off the couch and onto the floor." They were trying out an emerging trend that had been kicked off by the Beatles and the Maharishi Mahesh Yogi. She became Canada's echo to the 1960s wave of hippiedom and counterculture birthed in Haight-Ashbury in San Francisco. It was a movement whose time had come, and it needed a catalyst. Kareen was the right lady at the right time with the right message. Her life had prepared her for this mission.

Kareen was born in Germany to a temperamental mother and a brilliant physician father. He insisted Kareen attend a private school in Heidelberg, and made sacrifices for her to do so. Kareen describes her mother as an admirable, but rather difficult woman who had suffered emotionally due to her experiences in both World War I and II. Eventually, she left the marriage and immigrated to Canada, taking Kareen with her.

Kareen arrived in the small northern town of Dawson Creek, British Columbia, a considerable culture shock after Heidelberg. Her parents had instilled in her an unusually strong work ethic; thus, she was encouraged to study hard and skipped two grades to fit into the existing curriculum. During this time, she joined the drama club and learned writing skills.

All of these things were to serve her well in the future. Perhaps she was already sensing that more lay ahead.

When Kareen and her mother moved to Vancouver, Kareen enrolled in a Russian language class at the University of British Columbia. This is where she met her husband-to-be, Peter Zebroff. She describes it as "a *coup de foudre*—a lightning-bolt hit us both." They were married in 1961.

Peter relocated several times, first as a teacher and then as a principal. When he accepted a position in Hudson's Hope, British Columbia, Kareen began to feel increasingly isolated and became depressed and overweight. Her mother had taken yoga at Utica University (New York) while visiting Kareen's youngest sister there. It was so effective in giving her relief from menopausal problems that she highly recommended it to Kareen, who had admitted to feeling "down and dumpy." Kareen found the one and only book available on yoga in the general store, *Yoga, Youth and Reincarnation,* written by Jess Stearn, with poses modelled by the sagacious Marcia Moore.

From then on, Kareen's yoga practice was constant. She claims that the regular practice of yoga and meditation kept her sane while at home with her three little girls—all born within four years. Still, she felt something was missing in her life and "calling" to her. Kareen found it the next year when she approached continuing education officials about teaching yoga in the school gym near their new home in Agassiz, British Columbia. Skeptical, they said she had to get together at least ten people, adding "that just never happens" in their small town.

This fired Kareen up to write an article in the local newspaper, listing all the numerous benefits she had received practicing yoga. The result: seventy-four people stepped up and paid! Yoga's time had come! Soon, she was teaching three classes a week to the people of Harrison Hot Springs.

The launch of her TV show happened quite by chance.

The Harrison Hot Springs Hotel manager wanted her to help out in a "weight-loss week" through diet, exercise, and yoga. To promote this, the assistant manager, chef, and Kareen went onto a well-known afternoon CTV talk show and she stood on her head and talked. The next day, a surprised Kareen got a call from the director of programming saying that they happened to be working on a yoga pilot project with four applicants already lined up to host it. Would she like to audition? Would she?!

Kareen showed up the next afternoon in a ballet-type exercise suit she had bought that morning in a Vancouver dance supply store, with a cat in a basket, the Beatles' "Hey Jude" as intro music, a detailed lesson plan on cue cards. The rest, as they say, is history.

Kareen went on to film an impressive 1,100 daily half hour shows. She catapulted to fame in British Columbia within six months and then across Canada.

Her practical, spiral-bound book, *The ABC of Yoga*, topped over one million copies in sales in Canada and Germany—an exceptional number for its time.

The TV series' far-reaching success included rural and northern areas where no yoga teachers existed. Bringing yoga into isolated areas aroused a curiosity for yoga's physical, mental, and spiritual health benefits.

Kareen studied various topics both for her own healing and for sharing with her fans. Thus, her show format also had a guest-interview segment, and her "word of wisdom" at the end. The guest interviews were with notable experts in their fields, such as the famed Indra Devi, the well-known American yogini, hypnotherapist, and astrologer Marcia Moore (who had by then become her close friend and mentor), doctors, psychiatrists, chiropractors, nutrition book authors, ministers, rabbis, psychologists, as well as swamis like her own guru, Swami Shyam Acharya, Swami Vishnudevananda, and other esteemed yogis. As Kareen said: "We were like free-wheeling hippies back then, and we tried everything."

When she interviewed Swami Vishnudevananda, a strong advocate of vegetarianism, she opened up a topic that people were very curious about. Her international cuisine cookbook soon followed. Co-authored by vegetarian Pegge Gabbott, *Nutritious*

Recipes from Kareen's Kitchen sold over 25,000 copies in Canada alone.

By now, Kareen was receiving 1,000 letters per day from across Canada and the northern United States. Astonishingly, no publisher was interested in her book, so Peter started a publishing company for Kareen's nine books, some of which were published in eleven languages—Fforbez Enterprises was born.

Peter was Kareen's most stalwart supporter. Born of pacifist Russian Doukhobors in Grand Forks, British Columbia, his calm and easy nature proved to be her pillar of strength throughout her fame and during their fifty-eight years of marriage. He was her producer on TV, and he ensured that each of the 227,500 fan letters and book orders got a signed response.

Germany, too, was quick to claim one of its own. Kareen's father had seen her show while visiting Canada and urged her to try to do the same in Germany. During an appearance on Germany's most popular sport show, she demonstrated yoga poses and talked about the mystical aspects of yoga. Soon, she was flying there every three months to film for TV. Again, the timing had proved to be miraculously right for yoga. In January 1975, Kareen was the cover story of the prestigious *Der Spiegel* magazine and *The ABC of Yoga* hit Germany's bestseller list. Years later, she was to make another cover, that of the scholarly book *Yoga Traveling*, an interesting and unmatched academic account of the history of yoga in the world.

Kareen shared her personal evolution through yoga candidly with all who knew her. She dedicated herself to refining her intuitive powers and becoming a bit wiser about herself. She was experiencing profoundly altered states of consciousness with such yoga mystical states known as *kundalini* and *samadhi*, while meditating, at times all night, under the guidance of her guru, Swami Shyam Acharya, and others. Says Kareen: "The state of samadhi is devoutly to be wished for, as it is a 'bliss-consciousness.' During this experience there is a rare disembodiment—a detachment of mind from body, while floating rapturously in a kind of 'heaven.' I have experienced it at times, including at an opera, where the divine music of Mozart rained down upon me like a blessing."

Kareen learned to study and explore past-life regressions from her friend Marcia Moore, and she quietly admits that she consults daily with her own spirit-guides. "The answers, though sometimes surprising, are always about the 'truth' of the guides, not about yours," says Kareen. "Their messages are that love is what matters most, intent has no worth unless it is kind."

Kareen's contribution to yoga in Canada is unparalleled. If you shake the yoga tree, her influence is in every leaf. When asked to comment on that, Kareen states "I only showed up for the inevitable—that God and the universe work through us and with us when we are willing to allow it. The miracles look after them*selves*."

A private person, Kareen lives in Surrey, British Columbia, with her husband, Peter. Her passion is photography, writing two novels, and finishing her memoir.

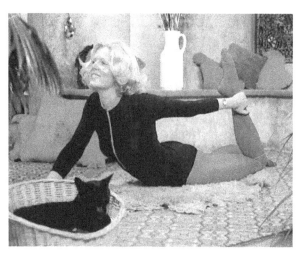

Kareen goes national with cat, *"Hey Jude,"*
and a gym suit

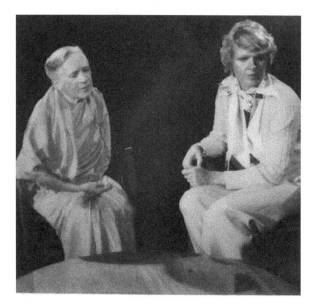

Kareen interviewing Indra Devi

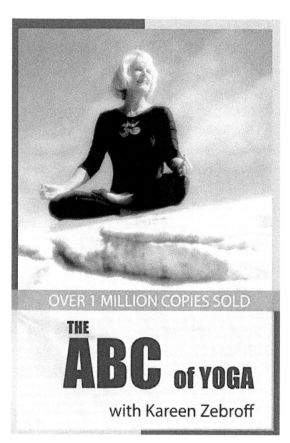

OVER 1 MILLION COPIES SOLD

THE
ABC of YOGA
with Kareen Zebroff

ABC, introducing yoga into Canadian homes

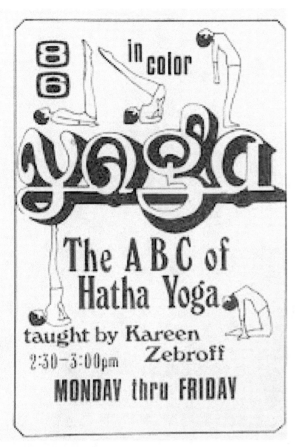

Early T.V. advertisement

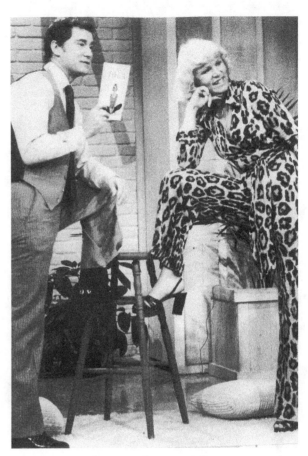

filming with Regis Philbin

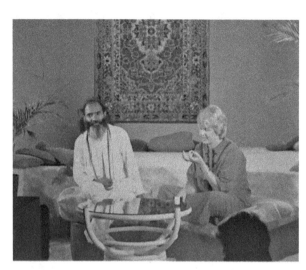

Kareen interviewing Swami Shyam Acharya, her
spiritual guide

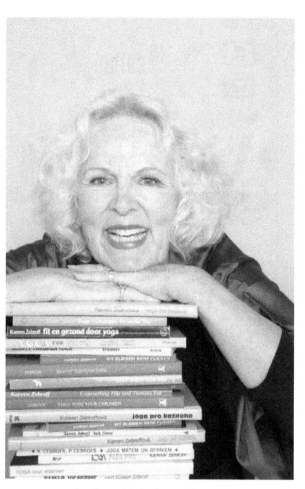

10 books published in 11 languages

Epilogue

At the time of this writing, several souls have slipped away silently, sadly, and all too quickly: Friedel Khattab, Marie Paulyn, Ruth Boutilier, Hilda Pezarro. I talked to their students, who felt grateful for what these teachers gave them—a practice in which to become fuller, more loving human beings as well as confidence to test the teachings and become their own spiritual pilgrims.

The initiatives launched by these individuals have now shaped a third generation of yoga practitioners and teachers. Predominantly female, they are reconciling a long-held tradition of guru lineage with their own ambitions, the resources to pursue them, and a vision of what can be. There is talk of co-sharing rather than being led through hierarchy. It is an interesting pivot in yoga history, an evolutionary page being turned. Shall we trust the process and let it reveal itself to us, as these pioneers did?

The frontiers these teachers opened seeped into Canadian culture. The business of yoga became acceptable. Yoga and meditation are now a complementary adjunct to physical therapy and psychotherapy and even different faith expressions. A frontier of energy as the new medicine is emerging, with these teachers being consulted for their wisdom on how subtle energies awaken in yoga practice. Studies continue on the relationship between yoga and aging as these seniors seem indefatigable and continue to inspire. There are many more not mentioned in this book. You don't have to look too far—they are glowing on a mat near you.

Yoga philosophy says time and distance mean little, that it is our thoughts and deeds that leave a karmic trail. If that is true, the lives of these exceptional people leave a legacy that speaks volumes: to pursue our intuitive hunches without fear, listen to the whispers from the infinite, heed the click that happens in our gut at opportune times, and trust the moments of synchronicity that point the way.

In reciting the echo chamber of OM, nature's tone-perfect primordial sound, we are reminded that we are all fleeting moments of vibration sharing the same stream of consciousness. As yoga philosophy teaches us, we are oneness without separation. We are consciousness seeking to realize itself to its fullest extent. To the degree that we become fulfilled, we avoid the bitter taste of regret. These teachers show us that it is truly in practice that we learn to abide in the Light, the *samadhi* of our existence, where science and spirituality exquisitely merge. We are OM.

Acknowledgements

Researching this book was a treasure hunt that took me to all kinds of unexpected places, accompanied by a spirit guide or two. The interviewees gave generously of their time as they rooted through a box in the garage, dusted off an old photograph, or otherwise provided bits and pieces in my search.

My deepest gratitude is to the illuminating people interviewed in this book. You believed teaching was its own reward, but your footprint is now a path. Your willingness to be authentic inspires many others, as was your courage in being unconventional.

My sincere thanks to the children and grandchildren who went down memory lane with me: Patrick Tomlinson, Jan Barylski, Virginia Anzlin, Penny Grant, Patricia Williams, David Bloom, Helene Paulyn, Heather Silberberg, and Sandra Silberberg.

To the spouses: Derek French for adding to the legacy of BKS Iyengar, Luella Sinha for sharing Ranen's memory, Jerry Boutilier for the heartfelt conversations when Ruth passed, and Christine Gnilke for sharing Joe's memories.

To Marie Oliver for her hospitality despite a New Brunswick flood rising almost to her front door! To Martha Schwartz and to Kerry Lawson for her friendship and vision To Neil Bixby, for his candor and insights. To Joyce Hawkeye, for her immaculate records. To Alan Trimble and Andrea (Lakshmi) Roth-Trimble, Josh McKay, Janet Siskund, Marion Harris, Bala Jaison, Wendy Cole and Paul Chaput. To Laurie Jo Lindroos and Susan Bull for their heartfelt support and wisdom.

To DeeDee Poyner for sharing the 1970s. To Jeannie Stevens for injecting her soul into the

Yukon and sharing her diaries and photos from those days.

To Swami Vijnananda (Yves Mayer) and Pauline Geoffrion for French interpretation. To Padmavati of the Sivananda Vedanta Yoga Centre

To Hari Singh Khalsa for sharing your life and the history of 3HO with me.

To Margaret Gupta for being the fairy godmother who filled in so many historical gaps at the eleventh hour.

To Kareen and Peter Zebroff, whose life experience and friendship flow throughout this book.

To Barb Thrasher and Larissa D'Silva for listening, proofing, and guiding and Rosemarie Bartschak for graphics.

To Debbie Spence, tireless stalwart of the Yoga Association of Alberta. To Carol Fedun, Chris Erdmann-Boyko, and Pam Chamberlain for helpful contributions.

To Swami Lalitananda for giving me unfettered access to archives at the Yasodhara Ashram and for her faith in me.

To Pam Patterson, Sandra Rose, and Dr. Stanley Brown for their support in regaling Bina Nelson.

To the YWCAs everywhere, who contributed so greatly to women's empowerment on our planet. Where would we be without you? Thanks to YWCA Vancouver, Toronto, and Victoria. Special mention to the YWCA Montreal residence, which has stood as a monumental bastion of hope for thousands since 1875 and who housed li'l ole me during my research.

To the helpful clerks at Public Archives Office, Charlottetown, PEI—there is no charm like PEI charm. To PEI's senior teacher today, Ruth Richmond, and to Rose and Fred Landrigan for sharing Laraine Crawford's memory.

To the archivists at the universities of Regina, Concordia, Alberta, Dalhousie, Toronto, British Columbia, Montreal, and Simon Fraser.

To Jools Andres, whose skills as a yoga therapist, writer, and editor helped me launch. To Jamie, Hayley, Jessica, Lucero and team at Friesen publishing for helping me get to the finish line.

To all my students, friends, and family who encouraged this project as worthwhile.

To my mom, who still gets on her mat every day at age eighty-five and who birthed my spiritual curiosity as my Sunday school teacher.

To my love, Tom, who lived with me and the book and believed in us both unflinchingly. Thank you. I owe you a hundred Indian dinners.

To my daughter Ivana, who was raised a high-performance athlete and became a Buddhist meditator. I love you. And I say to you and your generation, boldly meet the new frontiers. They await you.

Reading List

28 Day Exercise Plan, Richard Hittleman, 1972, Workman Publishing Co. New York, NY and 1995 Hamlyn Publishing, London, UK

The ABC of Yoga, Kareen Zebroff, 1971, published by Fforbez Enterprises Ltd.

Autobiography of a Yogi, Paramahansa Yogananda, 2016 Arcturus Publishing, London, UK or Crystal Clarity Publishers, Nevada City, CA

Bhagavad Gita, S. Radhakrishnan, 1973, Harper and Row, New York, NY, 2009, Vedanta Press, Hollywood CA (first published by Allen & Unwin, UK, in 1948. It has gone through several reprints, unchanged with them).

Beauty and Health through Yoga, 1980, Eve Diskin, Warner Book Publishing, New York, NY

Beauty through Yoga, Kareen Zebroff, 1989, published by Fforbez Enterprises Ltd.

The Chariot of Sadhana, Marion and Martin Jerry, 2006, Unlimited Publications, Bloomington, Indiana, 2M Communications, Canmore, Alberta

Compendium of Iyengar Yoga Practices—Special Needs, Marlene Mawhinney, 2013, published by Marlene Mawhinney

Compendium of Iyengar Yoga Practices—Special Practices, Marlene Mawhinney, 2013, published by Marlene Mawhinney

Diary of the Inner Teacher, Marion and Martin Jerry 2008, 2M publications, Canmore, Alberta

Complete Illustrated Book of Yoga, 1995, Swami Vishnudevananda, Harmony Publishing, New York, NY

Diary of the Inner Teacher, Marion and Martin Jerry 2008, 2M publications, Canmore, Alberta

Divine Light Invocation, Swami Radha, 2010, Timeless books, Kootenay Bay, BC

Encyclopedia of Indian Philosophies Vol. 12: by Gerald James Larson and Ram Shankar Bhattacharya 2011, published by Motilal Banarsidass Publishing, New Delhi, India

Fitness Through Yoga,1974, Hubert Dhanaraj, published by Hubert Dhanaraj, Edmonton, Alberta

40 Day Sadhana Manual, Marlene Mawhinney, 1987, published by Marlene Mawhinney, Toronto, Ontario

Journey to the Centre, Marion and Martin Jerry, 2016, 2M publications, Canmore, Alberta l

Kirtan: The Art and Ecstasy of Chanting, 2016, Divya Prabha, Shining Bay Books, Halifax, Nova Scotia

Kundalini Yoga for the West, Swami Radha, 2004, Timeless books, Kootenay Bay, British Columbia

Letters from the Masters, Mugs McConnell, 2016, published by North Atlantic Books, Berkeley, California

Light on Yoga, 2015, Harper Thorsons, New York, NY

Light on Life, 2006, Publishers: Potter/ Ten Spced/Harmony/Rodale

Light on Pranayama, BKS Iyengar, 2013, Thorsons Publishing

Light Sitting in Light, Sister Elaine MacInnes, 1997, published by Harper Collins, Toronto, Ontario

Mandukya Upanishad 2006, Swami Nikhilananda, published by Advaita Ashrama, Howrah, India

The Labyrinth of Solitude, Dadabhai Prithipaul, 2012, Coronet Books, London, UK, first published by Munshiram Manoharlal Publishers, New Delhi, 2002

Marlene Mawhinney, Iyengar Yoga Practices and The 40 Day Sadhana Manual, published by Marlene Mawhinney, Toronto, Ontario

Midwifing Distress at end of Life, Article by Karen Fletcher, 2013, Published in Palliative and

Supportive Care, Cambridge University Press, Cambridge, UK

Psoma Yoga Therapy, Donna Martin, 2020, Stones Throw Publications, Birmingham, UK

Remembering Wholeness, Donna Martin, 2002, Caribooklinks Publishing, Kamloops, British Columbia

Reincarnation: Key to Immortality, Marcia Moore, 1968, Arcane Publishing, London, UK

Science and the Sacred, 2002, Ravi Ravindra, Theosophical Publishing House, Adyar, Chennai India (directly from Ravi) Sutras of the Inner Teacher, Marion and Martin Jerry, 2001, Unlimited Publications, Bloomington Indiana, 2M Communications, Canmore, Alberta

The Sublime Myth of Rama, 2020, Dadabhai Prithipaul, Munshiram Manoharlal Publishers, New Delhi

Standing on a Platform of Kindness, Recording, Bev Zizzy, 2016, Regina, Saskatchewan

The Wisdom of Patanjalis Yoga Sutras: A New Translation and Guide, 2009, Ravi Ravindra, Morning Light Press, Sandpoint, Idaho (directly from Ravi)

Woman in Black, Recording, Bev Zizzy, 2009, Regina, Saskatchewan

Yoga Fiction, Yoga Truth, Sandra Sammartino, ebooks published 2014, White Rock, British Columbia

Yoga Fits In, Gerda Krebs, published by Gerda Krebs, 1978, Edmonton, Alberta

Yoga the Science of Self, 1979, Marcia Moore and Mark Douglas, Arcane Publications, London, UK

Yoga Self Taught, 1968, Andre Van Lysebeth, published by Flammarion Publishing, Paris, France (taken from Wikipedia)

Yoga and the Teaching of Krishna: Essays on the Indian Spiritual Traditions, Ravi Ravindra, 1998 Theosophical Publishing House, Adyar, Chennai India

Yogasutracintamani, Norman Sjoman, 2013, Black Lotus Books, Calgary, Alberta

Yoga: Two concepts and Four Choices, 1975, Ranendra Sinha, published University of Manitoba, Winnipeg, Manitoba

The Yoga Tradition of the Mysore Palace, 1996, Norman Sjoman, Black Lotus Books, Calgary, Alberta

Yoga Traveling: Bodily Practice in Transcultural
Perspective, 2013, Beatrix Hauser, Springer
International Publishing, Switzerland

Yoga, Youth and Reincarnation, Jesse Stearn, 1997,
Doubleday Books, Garden City, NY

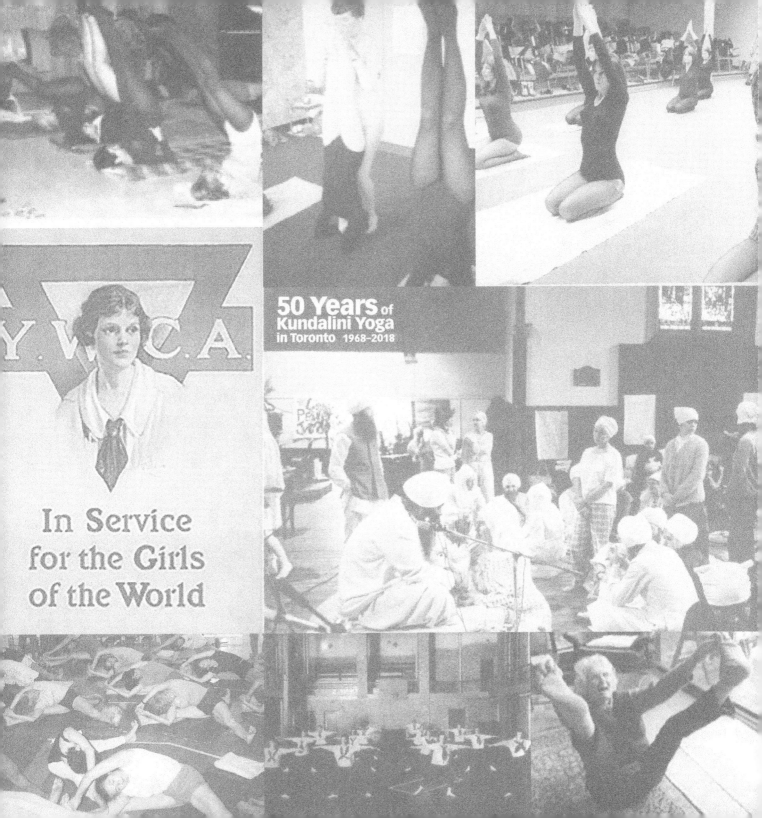

Y.W.C.A.

In Service
for the Girls
of the World

50 Years of
Kundalini Yoga
in Toronto 1968–2018

CPSIA information can be obtained
at www.ICGtesting.com
Printed in the USA
LVHW061501271022
731742LV00006B/353

9 781525 565236